SCC
$49.95

Caring for Muslim Patients

SECOND EDITION

Edited by

Aziz Sheikh MSc MD DCH DRCOG FRCGP FRCP
Professor of Primary Care Research & Development
University of Edinburgh, UK

Abdul Rashid Gatrad OBE PhD FRCP FRCPCH
Consultant Pacdiatrician, Manor Hospital, Walsall
Honorary Senior Lecturer, University of Birmingham, UK
Honorary Professor, University of Kentucky, USA

Foreword by
HRH The Prince of Wales

Radcliffe Publishing
Oxford • New York

Radcliffe Publishing Ltd
18 Marcham Road
Abingdon
Oxon OX14 1AA
United Kingdom

www.radcliffe-oxford.com
Electronic catalogue and worldwide online ordering facility.

First Edition 2000

British Library Cataloguing in Publication Data

A catalogue record for this book is available from the British Library.

ISBN-13: 978 1 85775 812 2

Typeset by Pindar New Zealand (Egan Reid) Auckland, New Zealand
Printed and bound by TJI Digital, Padstow, Cornwall, UK

Contents

Foreword to second edition

As we take our first steps into the twenty-first Century we face many challenges. One of the most pressing issues, I believe, is how we as a society manage to recognise and appreciate the importance of achieving a balance between our spiritual and physical needs. For, without this balance, I fear that modern medicine, despite all its breathtaking advances, will leave many people frustrated and confused.

It is my long-held belief that in this, as in other areas of life, the West has much to learn from the teachings of Islam. One of the most striking features of Muslim communities is the remarkable impact of the central grand narrative of Islam on the day-to-day lives of Muslims. Muslim respect for the spiritual as well as physical side of human life is particularly strong. The stability that such a framework brings is most evident during times of uncertainty and difficulty, like ill-health, loss and bereavement. This is, I believe, one reason why those charged with organising and delivering healthcare have to try to understand the needs and concerns of all religious groups.

Caring for Muslim Patients is an important first step in this task. Taking an 'insider's perspective', the book offers a useful insight into the British Muslim community. It should help healthcare professionals to understand the vocabulary and culture of this important sub-section of our community and, in so doing, provide clinicians with the tools needed to appreciate some of the concerns of this community. But the importance of this work extends beyond its aim to set out a rational basis to improve the delivery of healthcare to Muslims. It also provides new and valuable insights into ways in which notions of health and disease may be re-formulated so that the NHS and its highly skilled and dedicated staff are better equipped to appreciate the very many dimensions to healing.

HRH The Prince of Wales

Foreword to first edition

Three years ago I had the privilege of chairing a multifaith Working Party concerned with the healthcare needs of people from ethnic minorities in the United Kingdom. It quickly became clear that the outstanding need was for education of healthcare professionals to complement the enlightened initiatives being planned by the Department of Health. We conducted a survey of medical schools, which revealed that there was limited explicit or specific cross-cultural content in curricula at any stage. The Working Party made a number of appropriate recommendations. I should not be surprised if this book were to achieve more than my Working Party did in persuading healthcare professionals, and their teachers, of the need and value of cross-cultural education informed by an 'insider's feel'.

The National Health Service has a responsibility to provide healthcare for the whole population, with a focus on each unique individual. The message of this book is that both knowledge and insight are required to combat institutional racism, whether admitted or unconscious, and to cater positively for patients with a wide diversity of beliefs and practices in a multicultural society.

It was a shock to realise that although Muslims represent some 20% of the world's population, of whom almost two million are British citizens, and despite a Muslim presence in the United Kingdom stretching back hundreds of years, the rest of the population, including those responsible for their health and education, know little about the religion or its adherents. Ignorance is cause enough for concern; prejudice nurtured by stereotyped misconceptions and fostered by misrepresentation is worse by far. For example, the misconception that Islam is some kind of alien Eastern religion exclusively synonymous with Asia, or that it is a creed of intolerance and subversive fundamentalism which denigrates women, are fuelled by selective publicity given to those wretched 'Islamic' regimes whose oppressive power-hungry hierarchies can be seen as a blasphemy against 'the way of peace'.

Against this discouraging background, the authors could have been forgiven for penning a plaint against prejudice. Commendably, however, they seek to 'describe what it means to belong to a sacred tradition, to explore the intricate connections between faith and health for Muslims, and consider some of the implications of this relationship for those striving to deliver culturally competent and sensitive care'. Like the Muslim vision of the tripartite nature of man 'comprising spiritus, anima and corpus, and one in which unity reigns supreme', this book falls into three interwoven parts: an overview of Islam and its adherents, with particular reference to the United Kingdom; the Muslim patient on the earthly sojourn from birth to death; and informative appendices, including a full glossary. Throughout, the hallmarks of this 'exploration of the interface between faith and health' are restraint of expression and balance of content.

Believers in any faith, for whom life is sacred and living a sacred trust – notably the monotheistic religions – will revel in the contemplation of parallels, the similarities and differences between their beliefs and those expressed in this work. The elegant and scholarly text is a joy to read; as revelation succeeds revelation preconceptions are challenged, misconceptions are aborted, and the dawn of enlightenment stirs conviction that believers and non-believers alike must do what they can to respond as fellow human beings, especially those with the privileged responsibility of a doctor or other healthcare professional. In an increasingly secular society, whose traditional values nevertheless continue to be based upon its Judeo-Christian heritage, this work might well form a model for revisiting the relationship between faith and health for those older siblings of Islam.

The Editors sound a valedictory challenge to the more cynical reader when they write, 'evidence points in favour of religious practice being associated with a diverse array of health benefits, such as better obstetric outcome, lower blood pressure, reduced risk of cancer and increased overall life expectancy'.

And peace of mind?

Sir Alexander Macara
February 2000

About the editors

Professor Aziz Sheikh BSc MSc MD DCH DRCOG FRCGP FRCP was trained at University College, London and then undertook postgraduate studies at Northwick Park Hospital and the London School of Hygiene and Tropical Medicine. He is Professor of Primary Care Research and Development in the University of Edinburgh's Division of Community Health Sciences, co-chair of the Science and Research Committee of the British Thoracic Society, chair of the Diversity and Equalities Board of the National Clinical Assessment Service, research advisor to Education for Health, and GP editorial advisor to the *British Medical Journal*. He has co-authored/edited four multidisciplinary texts and has published over 300 papers in peer refereed journals. Aziz is blessed with four young children who take up most of his spare time.

Professor Abdul Rashid Gatrad OBE PhD FRCP FRCPCH was born in Malawi, Central Africa. He was educated in Zimbabwe, Harrow and then University of Leeds, UK. His postgraduate training was in the Manchester area. He is a Consultant Paediatrician at the Manor Hospital in Walsall, Hon Senior Lecturer at the University of Birmingham and Professor of Pediatrics (University of Kentucky, USA). He was the clinical postgraduate tutor at the Manor Hospital. He is an examiner to the Royal College of Paediatrics and sits on their Ethics Committee. He has published over 50 papers and co-authored two books. He has built an orphanage which he now runs in North West India and is actively involved in sending usable discarded medical equipment to Third World countries through a registered charity – the International Hospital Equipment Trust.

List of contributors

Abdul Aziz Ahmed Learning Support Manager, Glasgow.

Saddaf Alam General Practitioner, Oldham; Executive Committee, Mediconcern; and Member, Health and Medical Committee, Muslim Council of Britain.

Muhammad Anwar Research Professor, Centre for Research in Ethnic Relations, University of Warwick, Coventry.

Sangeeta Dhami Locum General Practitioner, Edinburgh.

Abdul Rashid Gatrad Consultant Paediatrician, Manor Hospital, Walsall; Honorary Senior Lecturer, Birmingham University, Birmingham; and Honorary Professor, University of Kentucky, USA.

Hamza Yusuf Hanson Director, Zaytuna Institute, California, USA.

Sir Alexander Macara Chairman of the UK Public Health Medicine Consultative Committee, and former Chairman of the British Medical Association Council.

Ahmed Sadiq Consultant Ophthalmic Surgeon, Manchester Royal Eye Hospital, Manchester.

Aziz Sheikh Professor of Primary Care Research and Development, Division of Community Health Sciences, University of Edinburgh, Edinburgh.

Tim J Winter Sheikh Zayed Lecturer in Islamic Studies, School of Divinity, University of Cambridge, Cambridge; and Director, Anglo-Islamic Institute.

Acknowledgements

We owe numerous debts – spiritual, material, intellectual and emotional – to the very many people who have contributed to our understanding of the ideas discussed in this work. The debts owed to these individuals we gratefully acknowledge, and we hope that through the pages that follow, they will recognise some of the fruits of their labour, energies, vision, encouragement and support.

Co-ordinating the production of a multi-author work involves considerable co-operation between the editors, contributors, referees and publishers. Our co-authors, chosen primarily because of their in-depth involvement and understanding of the day-to-day affairs of their Muslim community, took precious time away from their busy professional, social and family commitments to attend to our demands, and also in many instances to review the work of their fellow contributors. Many others have very kindly reviewed, commented and, through their suggestions and criticisms, improved upon earlier drafts of chapters. Though far too many to mention individually, we would in particular like to thank: Professor Richard Ashcroft, Dr Jane Bradley, Dr Brian Briggs, Gloria Daley, Suma Din, Professor George Freeman, Professor Geri-Ann Galanti, Asad Hamid, Dr Sarah Hartley, Professor Brian Hurwitz, Riffat Islam, Lesley-Anne Pratchett, Dr John Salinsky, Dr Iftikhar Saraf, Dr Sarah Scambler and Abdulla Trevathan. The first edition of this work was reviewed in numerous journals and having had the opportunity to study the thoughtful critiques offered by these reviewers has also helped us improve this work: to the editors of these journals and their reviewers, our thanks. Our publishers, Radcliffe Publishing, have also been extremely supportive and efficient throughout the long gestation period of this book and to them also we extend our gratitude.

Much of our contribution has been made in that prized period of time between work and sleep, at weekends and during vacations. To our families, immediate and extended, we express our heartfelt gratitude for not only have they patiently coped with our divided attentions but also they have, in every sense, supported, encouraged and shared in our endeavours. Ultimately we recognise that *All praise is for Allah, Lord of all the Worlds.*

When you were born, everyone was smiling
but you were crying.
Live such a life that, when you depart, everyone is weeping
but you are smiling.

– *Sa'di of Shiraz* (d. 1292)

Introduction

As practitioners who live and work in areas with significant Muslim communities – *of which we are a part* – it is clear that much can be done to improve the experience of healthcare for Muslim patients. Most important of all, we believe, is the recognition that patients, irrespective of their religious or cultural affiliation, have a right to be *heard*, and their perspectives and world-view respected. *Caring for Muslims* has been written to begin to address these concerns. It seeks to describe what it means to belong to a sacred tradition, to explore the intricate connections between faith and health for Muslims, and consider some of the implications of this relationship for those striving to deliver culturally competent and sensitive healthcare.

Some 50 years after the introduction of state-run and managed health care systems, arguably one of our most humane institutions, it is noteworthy that health providers in Europe and North America have found it difficult to adapt to the needs of minority groups. Created historically to serve the needs of White, culturally homogeneous populations, they now face the challenge of catering for the tapestry of beliefs and cultures found in pluralist societies. Minority groups in the West have traditionally been thought of in terms of race and, more recently, ethnicity, and there is now an important body of research and literature devoted to understanding the health needs of the principal ethnic groups. While such a framework has proved extremely useful, it is, however, inadequate to describe fully the richness and complexity of most modern pluralist societies. We are beginning to understand the strong association between deprivation and ill health, for example. It is now clear that the 'deprived' have particular health needs that need to be realised and addressed. Another important framework for seeking to understand individuals and communities is on the basis of creed or religious affiliation. This was recognised by The European Convention of Human Rights in 1950, when it sought to guarantee individuals 'the right to freedom of thought, conscience, and religion' and has been reiterated in the Human Rights Act (2000). That religious affiliation can affect perspectives on health, access to healthcare, and the quality and quantity of healthcare received, is slowly being recognised by those trained in the secular biomedical model.

There has existed a Muslim presence in the West for well over a millennium, yet despite this lengthy interaction, Islam unfortunately remains something of an enigma. The stereotype that Islam is a faith of intolerance, terrorism and fundamentalism abound in the popular press and has in recent times been given additional credence by a vile and vociferous 'Muslim' fringe. It is also surprisingly common for those involved with health policy and delivery to think of Muslims as synonymous with Asians and/or Arabs. Positions such as these reflect a profound misunderstanding of Muslims and Muslim society. Muslim numbers globally are estimated to exceed 1.2 billion, with communities found in each and every country. It is then a matter of some importance to understand and appreciate the values and beliefs of so large and influential a segment of the human race, and the estimated 19 million who have made their homes in the West. From our personal experiences, both as the providers and recipients of care, we can say with confidence that such understanding and appreciation is crucial to *connecting* and the interrelated notions of empathy, trust and respect.

Western Muslim communities are heterogeneous in many respects – in terms of dress, diet, language and ethnic origin. Such diversity is recognised and indeed encouraged in Muslim culture since *true diversity* is considered an affirmation of the Divine. The contributors to this book, raised in different world continents, representing different genders, cultures and generations, begin to reflect this diversity. What unites these peoples is a central narrative – an outlook and framework that permeates and colours all aspects of their being. The faith that Muslims profess is simple, yet is one that has given birth to a history that is as rich and complex as any. A failure to recognise this narrative makes it difficult for one to understand the Muslim, since even the rejection of religion in such peoples must be understood from within their cultural milieu.

Caring for Muslims begins with a discussion on the pattern and process of contemporary Muslim migration to the West, information that is essential to understanding the current demographies of these communities (Chapter 1). Through using Britain as a case study and highlighting the difficulties posed by deprivation, racial and religious discrimination, Anwar identifies important barriers that need to be overcome to promote the social, economic and political integration of Muslims and the Muslim way of life. Winter (Chapter 2) articulates the narrative within which Muslims live and seeks to understand the continued appeal of such an all-embracing doctrine in the face of the otherwise almost relentless march of secularism. There then follows a reflection on notions of health and ill health from within traditional Muslim culture, and in particular on the intricate relationship between faith and health (Chapter 3). The first section of this work concludes with Hanson considering some of the main principles underpinning Islamic bioethics and its application in the context of healthcare planning and provision (Chapter 4).

Section 2 focuses on issues of direct relevance to patient care. An array of subjects are discussed ranging from challenges facing the contemporary Muslim family (Chapter 5), to birth and death customs (Chapters 6 and 9), and to those relating to periods of particular significance in the Muslim calendar such as the times of fasting (Chapter 7) and pilgrimage (Chapter 8). Peppered with anecdote and clinical cases, representing but a small proportion of the tales and experiences that now form part of our travelogues, contributors have above all aimed to provide insight – an *insider's feel* – in the belief and hope that understanding is perhaps the key ingredient for empathy.

Our conclusions are presented in Chapter 10, seeking to place this work in the context of broader historical and social discussions about the rich, complex and intriguing interface between religion, health and healthcare provision. The appendices that follow are designed to provide practical assistance to those involved in the day-to-day care of Muslims, and as a resource for those interested in gaining a broader understanding of Muslim culture.

This work in no way exhausts the subject at hand; rather it should be seen as introductory and exploratory. We have been at pains to avoid promoting a stereotypical 'recipe book' approach to viewing Muslims. On the contrary, we aim to provide a foundation to begin the process of experiential learning, and the cultural context and backdrop within which the very *individual* clinical encounter should be placed. It seeks to shed light on areas of positive medical practice in the hope that an awareness of such innovation will create a climate that promotes culturally competent care to flourish and gain wider professional acceptance. It discusses issues that we believe are frequently the cause of misunderstanding and discord between healthcare providers and their Muslim patients, and approaches are suggested that are likely to lead to delivery of more culturally sensitive healthcare. Despite its limitations this work in all probability represents the most comprehensive summary of issues concerning the care of Muslims living in the West to date.

If the work presented here can go some way towards promoting more open, inclusive and informed dialogue about the interface between faith and health, we will have begun to discharge some of our debts. These debts we owe to those patients, colleagues and friends who, often unwittingly, whether in the consulting room, in hospital corridors, at workshops, in mosques or at family gatherings, shared with us their stories and experiences, and in so doing have served as the real inspiration for this book.

Aziz Sheikh and Abdul Rashid Gatrad
October 2007

Islam and Muslims – An Overview

CHAPTER 1

Muslims in the West: demographic and socio-economic position

☾★ *Muhammad Anwar*

There are estimated to be 1.2 billion Muslims in the world, approximately one-third of whom live as religious minority communities. The largest minority Muslim community is to be found in India, where numbers of Muslims are estimated at about 140 million. A significant and growing number of Muslims are now also resident in the West. Approximately 60% of the 19 million or so Muslims living in the West are to be found in Western Europe, the rest living mainly in the United States (US), Canada and Australia, with small numbers in other Western countries. Though disparate, Muslims in the West face certain common issues as minorities in the countries of their residence, these including the fact that they are relatively young communities and thus typically have poorly developed infrastructures, and experience discrimination and political marginalisation. In this chapter I present a brief overview of Muslims in the West, concentrating in particular on Muslims in the US and in Western Europe. Then, by using Britain as a case study, I describe the pattern and process of migration, outline the demographic characteristics and examine the social, economic, political and health status of British Muslims. This in-depth case study of British Muslims should help to throw a much needed light on the situation of Muslims in the West.

Muslims in the West

The presence of Muslims in the West can be traced back to almost the beginning of Islam. For example, Muslims were in Spain and Sicily from the 8th to the 15th centuries. Muslim Tatars were in the Volga Valley from the 12th century and the Ottoman Empire's expansion into Europe took place in the 15th and 16th centuries. These periods brought Muslims to Western Europe in significant numbers.

The earliest Muslims to arrive in America in sizeable numbers came from West Africa as slaves between 1530 and 1851. They comprised an estimated 14–20% of the hundreds of thousands of West African slaves removed from their homelands.[1]

There were two waves of Muslim migration to the West in the 20th century that are important to mention. The first was after World War I and towards the end of the Ottoman Empire when Muslims from Syria, Lebanon and other Arab countries migrated to the US in large numbers.[1] The second wave, after World War II, included a significant number of Muslims migrating from all parts of the Muslim world to the West. These were mainly economic migrants either from former colonies such as Algerians to France, Pakistanis to Britain, Indonesians to the Netherlands, or were specially recruited to meet the economic and labour needs of the West as in the case of Germany, the US, Canada and Australia. Muslims in the West also include a growing number of those who converted to Islam in the last few decades such as African Americans and White Europeans. Table 1.1 gives an estimate of the number of Muslims now living in the West.

TABLE 1.1 Muslim population in the West: Estimates

COUNTRY	NUMBER OF MUSLIMS (MILLIONS)
US	6.0
Canada	0.6
Australia	0.4
Germany	3.1
France	4.0
Britain	1.8
The Netherlands	0.6
Belgium	0.5
Spain	0.4
Italy	0.5
Sweden, Denmark and Norway	0.3
Rest of Western Europe	0.7
Total	18.9

Source: This table is prepared by using various latest estimates. In particular, see M. Anwar 'Muslims in Western Europe: Responses to Integration', in T. Miyajima, T. Kajita and M. Yamada (eds), *Regionalism and Immigration in the Context of European Integration*, Osaka, The Japan Center for Area Studies, 1999.

Muslims in the United States, Canada and Australia
United States

Muslims in the US have diverse ethnic and national backgrounds. It is estimated that over 25% are African American and just over 24% are from India, Bangladesh and Pakistan; a further 27% are categorised as Arabs. The rest (24%) are from Iran, South Asia, and other smaller groups including 1.6% White American Muslims.[2] Like Muslims in Western Europe, they are highly concentrated in certain areas. Almost half of American Muslims live in 10 states: California (1 000 000), New York (800 000), Illinois (400 000), Indiana (180 000) and Michigan (170 000). It is estimated that there are 2000 mosques in the US, compared with 600 in 1980, 230 in 1960 and only 19 in 1930.[3] In addition, there are 400 Islamic schools (of which 108 are full-time) and more than 400 Muslim associations.

Because of the selective migration policy of the US in the 1960s and 1970s, which favoured mainly educated and professional people, the position of US Muslims in the labour market is quite good. But those who have migrated since the 1973 oil crisis have a comparatively lower socio-economic status and typically undertake unskilled and unsocial jobs such as working in restaurants and driving taxis.

Muslim households are larger than the national average, which reflects the younger population. On the whole, there are more Muslim poor families in terms of income than the national average in the US.[4] The general socio-economic situation of American Muslims, with particular reference to civil rights, is monitored by the Council on American-Islamic Relations (CAIR). In its 2001 report, it noted that American Muslims complained about the lack of accommodation in the workplace and schools. *Hijab* (headscarf) related complaints were among the most numerous. In the workplace, Muslims were often pressured to compromise their faith. The consideration of Muslim students' religious requirements within the public schools varied from one district to another.[5] It was also reported that Muslim employees in professional occupations often complained about difficulties in securing job promotion. Muslim college students complained that their freedom of speech had been violated and that Islam was misrepresented in the textbooks chosen by schools and instructors.[5]

There were also criticisms of the 1996 anti-terrorism law which was used almost exclusively against Muslims. Overall, it appears that discrimination is now part of daily life for American Muslims and since 11 September 2001 backlash hate crimes against Muslims have increased significantly.[6] It is, however, important to note that public officials have taken steps to minimise such violence, to ensure its successful investigation and prosecution, and to reassure Muslims that the government is committed to their protection.[6]

Canada

The Muslim presence in Canada is not new – the first mosque was officially opened in Alberta in 1938, this being built by the children of Muslim farmers and fur traders. The number of Muslims in Canada has increased substantially in recent years, increasing from 293 000 in 1991 to the present figure of about 650 000. Over 50% of Muslims are Canadian-born, and almost 3% of these Canadian Muslims are converts. The Muslim population is highly concentrated, particularly in Toronto. The number of mosques has risen significantly and there are many Muslim schools; for example, there are 16 in Toronto alone. Because of selective migration policies the socio-economic position of Muslims is quite good. For example, Muslims are better educated than most Canadians; 27% have graduate degrees as compared to 17% of all other Canadians.[7] Their contributions as pioneering farmers in Alberta, and in industry, government and high-tech enterprises are well recognised. However, since the 11 September 2001 tragedy in the US, attitudes towards Muslims have become more hostile. One poll in November 2002 of 1400 Canadians found that 44% of people were in favour of restricting the number of Muslims migrating to Canada.[8]

Australia

The 1996 Australian census showed that there were 200 885 Muslims in the country. However, recent estimates show that there are about 400 000 Muslims in Australia, of whom more than one-third are Australian born. Muslims are mainly concentrated in the states of New South Wales and Victoria. Australia's first mosque was built in 1861, and there are now 100 mosques in the country and over 20 Muslim schools. The Australian Federation of Islam Councils is the national body which represents over 100 community organisations. Muslims continue to make an important contribution to the socio-economic life of Australia and this is acknowledged by the government. The climate, however, changed somewhat following the 2002 Bali bombing in which many Australians were killed and there have been attacks on Australian mosques and reports of increasing hostility towards Muslims. There have also been problems in terms of local government attitudes to Muslims and negative media coverage of Islam and Muslims.[9]

Muslims in Western Europe

Most first generation Muslims who migrated to Western Europe after World War II left their countries of origin to find work with higher wages, hoping to accumulate savings with which to return to their countries after a few years. With changes in immigration policies in Western Europe, however, there has been a tendency for them to settle permanently, and the myth of return has gradually diminished.[10]

The majority of Muslims in Western Europe came from Turkey, Algeria, Morocco, Tunisia, Pakistan, Bangladesh, India, the Arab countries, the former Yugoslavia and in smaller numbers from several Third World Muslim and non-Muslim countries. There are many reasons for the migration of Muslims to Western Europe, the most common of which can be grouped under 'pull' factors, such as new job opportunities and economic prosperity, which attracted

Muslims to certain European countries, and the 'push' factors, like higher unemployment and underdevelopment, which forced them to leave their countries of origin. There is now no significant 'primary' immigration taking place into Western Europe.

In Britain, France and the Netherlands, colonial links and relevant rules about the admission of colonial subjects helped in the 1950s and 1960s the flow of migration from such ex-colonies as India, Pakistan, Bangladesh, Algeria, Indonesia, the West Indies and Surinam. However, later restrictions were introduced to discourage the free flow of people to their 'motherlands'. The migration of Muslims to Germany was, in contrast to many other countries, highly organised,[11] particularly from Turkey. As a result, Turks are the largest Muslim community, with over two million, in Germany.

Like other post-war migrants, Muslims settled in industrial areas where job opportunities were most available. Active kinship and friendship networks and the process of chain migration have contributed to the subsequent concentrations of Muslims in particular regions and cities.[10]

Research shows that Muslims in Western Europe have particularly acute problems, some of which relate to their legal and social status, some of which they share in common with other ethnic minorities and migrants. Others relate to their religion, languages, values and customs to which many feel that aspects of Western culture are a threat. Hence, they have a tendency to be conservative and protective. Hostility and discrimination from the indigenous people prompt Muslims to seek support from their own communities. They are sometimes blamed for the ills of the societies in which they live, such as high unemployment. However, the reality is that they are often the victims of these ills. Because of their young age profile and their willingness to undertake the low paid and unpopular jobs that indigenous workers are often unwilling to do, they are making a considerable contribution to the economies of Western Europe. But, despite this, both first generation migrant Muslims and their children continue to experience disproportionately higher unemployment rates when compared with White people from the same areas. This is partly due to the fact that many Muslims achieve poorly at school and therefore find it increasingly difficult to find work in an ever-shrinking manual/unskilled job market, but also because of racial and religious discrimination. Furthermore, many Muslims face language difficulties which hinder, in part, their progress in the industrial and social sectors. For example, Muslim workers are largely confined to unskilled jobs and work in 'minority ethnic group' situations where they often work unsocial night shifts and as a result have limited opportunities for communication with indigenous workers or mainstream society. These problems faced by Muslims are also relevant to the health services in the countries of their residence.

After these initial general comments on Muslims in North America, Australia and Western Europe, I now focus in detail on some of the issues raised through a case study of British Muslims.

Case study of British Muslims

Muslims are now an integral part of multiracial, multicultural and multifaith Western Europe and they form the largest religious minority group. A significant number have migrated to Britain in the last 50 years; their presence in this country, however, is not new.[12] The first mosque, for example, was established in Woking in 1890. Discussions on the well-established association between poverty and ill health fall beyond the scope of this case study and will therefore not be considered. Interested readers are referred to the reports of the two independent inquiries on health inequalities commissioned by recent Conservative and Labour governments.[13,14]

Migration and the myth of return

The large-scale Muslim migration to Britain followed the conclusion of World War II. This process, as mentioned above, is perhaps best characterised in terms of the 'pull' factors which attracted Muslims to Britain, and the 'push' factors which forced them to leave their countries of origin.[15] The 'pull' factors included a combination of economic and social developments in Britain, during the early post-war years. A period of rapid and continuous economic growth resulted in new and upward employment opportunities for indigenous workers, particularly for those with strong educational backgrounds and specialist non-manual skills. Consequently, few indigenous workers were willing to do unskilled manual jobs or shift work, creating a labour shortage in these areas. 'Push' factors included high unemployment rates, underdevelopment and few economic opportunities in the Indian subcontinent, from where the majority of Muslim migrants trace their origins. For those migrating from countries of the New Commonwealth, there were no restrictions to enter Britain until 1962, thereby allowing mass migration.

The primary migration into Britain from these regions has now almost stopped and only the reunification of families (i.e. the entry of dependants) is allowed, although this too has been made very difficult.[16] What was intended as a temporary sojourn in the West has, for many reasons, resulted in a more permanent settlement.[10]

Demographic characteristics

Most British Muslims have either acquired British nationality or were born in Britain. They should therefore no longer be considered as 'immigrants', but rather as 'settlers'; as discussed above the same cannot be said of Muslims in some other countries of Western Europe. The largest number of British Muslims (about 750 000) originate from Pakistan, with sizeable groups from Bangladesh, India, Cyprus, Malaysia, Arab countries and some parts of Africa. In addition, there is a small but growing number of indigenous British Muslims who have converted to the faith.

The UK Census is the most comprehensive source of demographic, geo-graphical, social and economic information about the general population and ethnic minorities in Britain. Questions about ethnicity were first included in the 1991 Census, revealing an ethnic minority population that was just over 6% of the total British population. In the 2001 Census the ethnic minority population increased to almost 9% of the population as shown in Table 1.2. In 1991 respondents were asked to classify themselves into one of nine categories. However, in the 2001 Census these categories were increased to 16 (Table 1.2).

TABLE 1.2   Ethnic groups in the 2001 Census

ETHNIC GROUP	ENGLAND AND WALES %	ENGLAND %	WALES %
White			
British	87.5	87.5	96.0
Irish	1.2	1.3	0.6
Other White	2.6	2.7	1.3
Mixed			
White & Black Caribbean	0.5	0.5	0.2
White & Black African	0.2	0.2	0.1
White & Asian	0.4	0.4	0.2
Other Mixed	0.3	0.3	0.1
Asian or Asian British			
Indian	2.0	2.1	0.3
Pakistani	1.4	1.4	0.3
Bangladeshi	0.5	0.6	0.2
Other Asian	0.5	0.5	0.1
Black or Black British			
Caribbean	1.1	1.1	0.1
African	0.9	1.0	0.1
Other Black	0.2	0.2	0.0
Chinese	0.4	0.4	0.2
Other ethnic groups	0.4	0.4	0.2
All ethnic groups	100	100	100

Source: The 2001 Census.

For the first time the 2001 Census also included a voluntary question on religion. It asked, 'What is your religion?', offering the response options shown in Table 1.3. Although a voluntary question, completion rates were high (92%). Results from analysis of this question found that there were 1.6 million Muslims in Britain in 2001. Table 1.3 provides a religious breakdown of the population in England and Wales in 2001. It is estimated that numbers will reach just over two million by 2010.

TABLE 1.3 Religion in Britain in 2001

	THOUSANDS	%
Christian	42 079	71.6
Buddhist	152	0.3
Hindu	559	1.0
Jewish	267	0.5
Muslim	1 591	2.7
Sikh	336	0.6
Other religion	179	0.3
All religions	*45 163*	*76.8*
No religion	9 104	15.5
Not stated	4 289	7.3
All no religion/not stated	*13 626*	*23.2*
Base	*58 789*	*100*

Source: The 2001 Census.

Gender

Initially, the migration of Muslims was predominantly of males. The study of the changing male to female ratio for Pakistanis, the largest subgroup of Muslims, vividly depicts the changing structure of the British Muslim community. In 1961, for example, 82% of Pakistanis were males, while in 1982 this had dropped to only 58%. After gaining economic security, the male migrants arranged for their families to be reunified. The 2001 Census found that Muslims are the only religious group in which men outnumber women – 52% compared with 48% – but when put into the broader context the sex ratio is clearly moving towards that of the indigenous White community.

Age profile

As evident from Figure 1.1, the Muslim population in Britain is much younger on average than the general population. Of particular note are the high proportion of young people and the very low prevalence of those aged 65 or over. Over half of British Muslims are now British born.

Household size

It is clear from Figure 1.2 that Muslims have the largest average household size in Britain. Possible explanations for this finding include the strong religious ethic encouraging fecundity and the extended nature of the Muslim family (*see* Chapter 5).[17]

FIGURE 1.1 Age distribution by religion, 2001

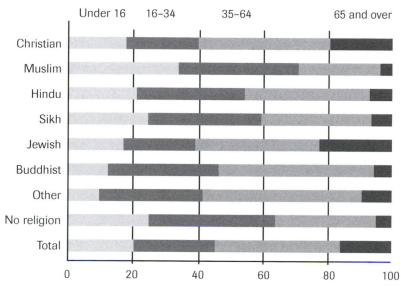

Source: The 2001 Census.

FIGURE 1.2 Average household size: by religion of household reference person, 2001

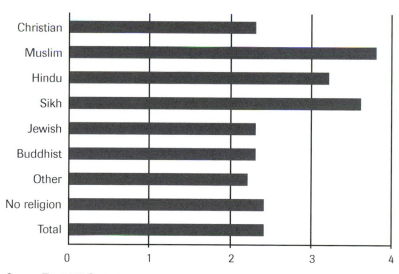

Source: The 2001 Census.

Geographical distribution

Like other post-war migrants, Muslims settled in industrial areas where employment opportunities were most promising. As mentioned above, active kinship, friendship networks and the process of chain migration have contributed to British Muslims concentrating in the former industrial strongholds.

The 2001 Census showed that 607 083 Muslims were living in London. Large communities are also found in the Midlands (191 559), West Yorkshire (149 689) and Greater Manchester (125 219). Birmingham in 2003, for example, had 150 000 Muslims, while Bradford's Muslim population was estimated to be 80 000.

Socio-economic position

Employment

Most first generation Muslim males were economic migrants to Britain. Consequently, their position in the labour market has determined, and continues to determine, their social standing both within their immediate family and in the wider community.

On arrival in Britain, Muslims had access to a limited range of occupations, most of which were either of an unskilled or semi-skilled manual variety. The demise of the industrial sector, coupled with the difficulties in finding alternative employment, led many to start their own businesses. The 1991 Census (for which no data by religion are available) showed that 24% of all employed Pakistanis and 19% of all employed Bangladeshis had their own businesses, compared with 13% of Whites. Of these, almost 40% of Pakistanis and over 70% of Bangladeshis were employers, making an additional valuable contribution to the economy through the creation of new employment opportunities. The most recent data from 2004 show that 18% of all Muslims in employment are self-employed compared with 13% of the general population. Though still very under-represented in managerial and professional positions, the emergence of a second generation British Muslim community, more versatile and better adapted to British institutions, has resulted in some diversification of employment patterns and this trend is likely to continue.

With respect to female employment, it is interesting to note that a much lower proportion of Muslim women are in employment when compared with White women. The 1991 Census showed the economic activity rate for Pakistani and Bangladeshi women to be low, 29% and 22% respectively, compared with 71% for White women, for example. These differences can largely be explained by religious teaching (*see* Chapter 5), but may in addition reflect employment disadvantages faced by Muslims and other minority groups in general and women in particular.

Evidence from the 1991 Census and Labour Force Surveys clearly showed that the unemployment rate for Muslim groups was almost three times as high as the

FIGURE 1.3 Unemployment rates: by religion and sex, 2004

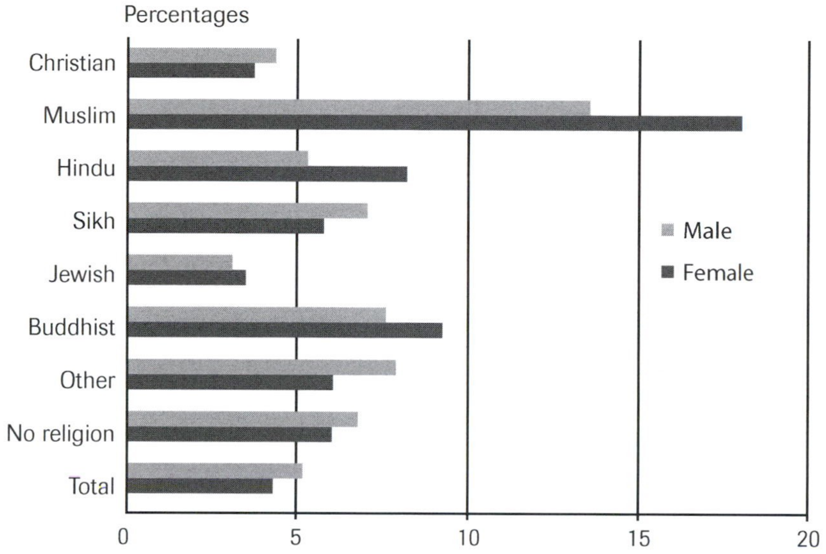

Percentages

[Bar chart showing unemployment rates by religion and sex. Categories from top to bottom: Christian, Muslim, Hindu, Sikh, Jewish, Buddhist, Other, No religion, Total. Each has Male and Female bars. Legend: Male, Female. X-axis scale: 0, 5, 10, 15, 20]

Source: Annual Population Survey, 2004.

rate for Whites and, as shown in Figure 1.3, more contemporaneous data show that this marked disadvantage persists. There is little doubt that discrimination against Muslims, and other minority groups, contributes to their high levels of unemployment. Of particular concern is that British born and educated Muslims appear to face the same disadvantages as did the first generation of Muslim migrants. A growing body of research indicates that this disadvantage is not confined to the lower-skilled jobs, but is also experienced when competing for well-respected professional vocations such as medicine and teaching,[18] indicating that discrimination is endemic within British society.

Housing

I have argued elsewhere that discrimination in employment has a magnifying effect on other important areas such as education and housing.[19] The location and quality of housing may in turn impact on the quality of overall health status. Data from the 2001 Census revealed that Muslim households were the most likely to be living in social rented accommodation, and are most likely to be living in overcrowded households (32% vs. 8% in the general population).

Education

Educational issues characteristically excite passionate discussion and debate within the Muslim community, largely on account of the prevalent belief that education offers perhaps the only avenue out of poverty. Research shows that Muslims fare worse in educational achievement than do White children.

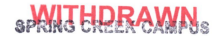

For example, I have found that Muslim children achieved lower General Certificate of Secondary Education (GCSE) examination results than did White children.[15] Geographical variations were noted, with Muslim children in Glasgow and some areas of London performing better on average than those in Birmingham and Bradford. Detailed analysis shows that these differences are attributable to social class and the duration of residence in Britain.

It is encouraging to see that an increasing number of Muslims are opting to pursue higher educational opportunities, despite the many biases operating against them. I have shown that there is a marked difference in acceptance rates to British universities between Muslims (40%) and Whites (54%) with identical qualifications.[15] Other educational issues considered to be important by Muslims include mother-tongue teaching, religious education, provision of *halal* (lawful) meals, prayer facilities, single-sex education and state funding of Muslim schools.[20] To help place this last issue in its correct context it is worth mentioning that although there are over 80 independent Muslim schools in Britain, only five of these have received state funding. In each of these cases this decision followed a long, and at times bitter, campaign involving Muslims the length and breadth of Britain. In contrast, there are several thousand Church of England, Catholic and Jewish schools that have voluntary-aided status and are in receipt of state funding.

Health status

There remains a dearth of data on health status by religion, but the 2001 Census data do offer some important insights. The Census asked two questions on health status: 'Over the last 12 months would you say your health has on the whole been Good, Fairly Good, Not Good'; and 'Do you have any long-term illness, health problem or disability which limits your activities or the work you can do?'

Figures 1.4 and 1.5 provide age-standardised responses to these questions and clearly show that Muslims fare worse than all other religious groups in relation to self-reported poor health and life-limiting illness/disability. Given these concerning findings, there is clearly a need to better understand why such inequalities exist and what steps can be taken to reduce them.

Community facilities and political participation

Muslims in Britain have responded well to meet the religious and cultural needs of their communities. An extensive network of community facilities now exists, ranging from mosques to youth and women's groups. In order to organise these facilities several local and regional organisations have been formed. Current estimates are that there are over 1200 local Muslim organisations and almost 1000 mosques. Many of these mosques are in makeshift premises, usually converted houses or factories, offering only the most basic facilities. The newer mosques, located within the major British cities, however, tend to be

FIGURE 1.4 Age-standardised 'not good' health rates: by religion and sex, 2001

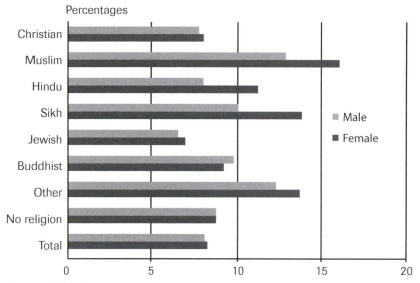

Source: The 2001 Census.

FIGURE 1.5 Age-standardised limiting long-term illness or disability rates: by religion and sex, 2001

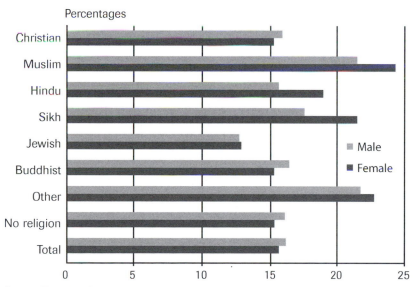

Source: The 2001 Census.

purpose-built, incorporating community halls and recreational facilities for young people. There are 58 mosques in Birmingham and nearly 50 mosques in Bradford, these figures giving some insight into the importance with which British Muslims view communal prayer facilities.

A more recent development has been the emergence of national co-ordinating agencies. The Union of Muslim Organisations in the United Kingdom and Eire (UMO) is one such organisation that operates primarily through lobbying central government on issues considered to be of importance to Muslims. The Muslim Council of Britain (MCB) was launched in November 1997 as a national umbrella group; it has a current membership of over 400 Muslim organisations. Other important organisations, albeit with a more limited remit, include the United Kingdom Islamic Mission, the Islamic Foundation, the Muslim Education Trust, the National Muslim Education Council of the UK and the Council of Mosques (for contact details *see* Appendix 2).

Mosques play an important educational role in teaching children the basic tenets of the Islamic faith as well as ensuring communal prayer facilities. Muslim organisations locally, regionally and now nationally provide an opportunity for the development of religious and cultural awareness in order to strengthen community ties. The same is true, to varying degrees, for Muslims in other Western European countries, as well as in the US, Canada and Australia, depending on the social and legal constraints imposed by their respective governments.

Most Muslims in Britain are entitled to vote and stand for elections both as British and/or as Commonwealth citizens. The willingness of Muslims to engage in the political process is increasing, but progress in translating this willingness into significant achievements has been slow. At a local level, there are now over 200 Muslim councillors. In the last European Parliament elections, two Muslims were elected MEPs, one to represent the British Conservative Party and the other to represent Liberal Democrats. The first Muslim MP, Mohammed Sarwar, was elected in the 1997 general election representing the Labour Party for the constituency of Glasgow Govan. He was joined in 2001 by Khalid Mahmood, (representing Birmingham Perry Barr), and in 2005 by Sadiq Khan (representing Tooting) and Shahid Malik (representing Dewsbury), all representing the Labour Party. However, there need to be at least 20 Muslim MPs to reflect accurately the size of the British Muslim community. In recent elections in Scotland and Wales, for the first time a Muslim was elected to the Scottish Parliament to represent the Scottish National Party (SNP) and another Muslim was elected to the Welsh Assembly to represent Plaid Cymru (PC).

Seven individuals of Muslim origin have recently been appointed as life peers in the House of Lords, four to represent the Labour Party, but again this figure needs to increase quite markedly. The representation of Muslims on public bodies is also very small. They are also under-represented in the civil service, the armed forces, the police, judiciary and other key appointments. Considering medicine, for example, it is regrettable to note that there has never been a Muslim president of one of the Royal Colleges.

Insecurity and identity

In 1997, the report by the Runnymede Trust Commission on British Muslims and Islamophobia[21] concluded that Muslims in Britain face religious discrimination and prejudice on an almost daily basis, contributing significantly to the insecurity complained of by so many. Among other things, the report draws attention to the stereotypical way in which Muslims are portrayed in the popular media as either 'terrorists' or 'fundamentalists', and the vulnerability of Muslims to physical violence and harassment. Muslims residing in many other Western European countries, such as France and Germany as well as in the US, also experience this phenomenon. The Rushdie affair, the Gulf War, the genocide of Muslims in Bosnia, the war in Afghanistan and the 11 September 2001 and 7 July 2005 attacks on the US and UK respectively have further contributed to this sense of vulnerability and alienation lamented on frequently by Muslims throughout the West.

The children of first-wave Muslim migrants represent a generation caught between two cultures. They live in the culture of their parents at home, but are often taught a different set of values and norms in schools, at work and through the media. Their world is not the 'old' or the 'new', but rather 'both'.[22] The process of acculturation, more marked in the youth, inevitably results in dissonance and disagreement at times between parents and their children. Thus, while the typical response of first generation Muslims to racial taunts, or physical violence, would be an acceptance of the situation, the same cannot be said of their children. On the contrary, they can at times be heard chastising their parents on account of their passivity, arguing that a failure to respond has allowed such wrongs to continue as was demonstrated in street disturbances in Oldham, Burnley and Bradford in the summer of 2001. It is my belief that the second generation Muslims present the real test as to how far Islamic beliefs and practices will be sustained in a non-Islamic environment, raising questions surrounding the future identity of British Muslims. My research suggests that the commitment to the Islamic ethic and culture among this second generation of Muslims remains strong, though not always in exactly the same patterns of their parents.[22]

Summary

↦ Muslims in the West are now an integral part of their countries of residence. They come from diverse backgrounds and are organised in various communities with different legal and socio-economic status. Most are, however, still marginalised. For example, their high unemployment rates, lower income and poorer housing conditions, which are common among Muslims in Western Europe, are likely to contribute to differential patterns of ill health compared with other communities.

↦ Muslims form Britain's largest religious minority group. Numbers are currently estimated at around 1.8 million with a projected rise to just over

2 million by 2010. Their demography differs quite markedly from that of the indigenous White population, reflecting the process and pattern of migration to Britain. The British Muslim community has a high proportion of males and young people, and a very low proportion of elderly people.

⇢ Racial discrimination and religious discrimination (Islamophobia) are major concerns of the British Muslim community. Legislation outlawing racial discrimination has existed for over 40 years, yet despite this racism continues to blight the day-to-day life of minority groups. Religious discrimination, except in employment, is still not outlawed in Britain.

⇢ Community facilities are becoming better developed, these typically having a strong religious dimension. There is an extensive network of mosques and community groups that continue to play a central role in the life of these communities.

⇢ Second generation Muslims form the test case to determine the degree to which Muslims will sustain Islamic beliefs and practices in a secular environment. Initial impressions suggest that their commitment to Islam remains strong.

References

1 Queen EL, III, Prothero, SR and Shattuck G Jnr. (1996) *The Encyclopedia of American Religious History.* Facts on File: New York.

2 Zogby International (2000) Survey commissioned by the American Muslim Council quoted in US Department of State (2001) *Fact Sheet: Islam in the United States.* Washington; and Kahera AI (2002) Urban Enclaves, Muslim Identity and the Urban Mosque in America. *Journal of Muslim Minority Affairs,* **22**: No.2.

3 Khalidi O (2000) Mosque. In Roof WC (ed), *Contemporary Religion,* Macmillan: New York.

4 Kosmin B and Mayer E (2001) *American Religious Identification Survey 2001,* City University of New York.

5 Nimer M (2001 *The Status of Muslim Civil Rights in the United States,* Council on American-Islamic Relations: Washington.

6 Human Rights Watch (2002) '*We Are Not the Enemy': hate crime against Arabs, Muslims and those perceived to be Arab or Muslim after September 11*; **14**: No.6(G): New York.

7 *Muslims in Canada* see www.Islam.ca and Canadian Association of Islamic Relations (CAIR Canada) www.isnacanada.com/cair

8 Blanchfield M (21 December 2002) 'Keep Muslims out, poll says; nearly half of Canadians want immigration control', *The Times Colonist* (Victoria): Ottawa.

9 Australian Department of Foreign Affairs and Trade (2002) *Islam in Australia,* www.dfat.gov.au/facts/islam_in_australia.html Also see Saeed A and Akbarzadeh S (eds) (2001) *Muslim Communities in Australia.* University of New South Wales Press: Sydney.

10 Anwar M (1979) *The Myth of Return.* Heinemann: London.

11 Anwar M (1999) Muslims in Western Europe: Responses to Integration. In Miyajima T, Kajita T and Yamada M (eds) *Regionalism and Immigration in the Context of European Integration,* The Japan Center for Area Studies: Osaka.

12 Matter N (1998) *Islam in Britain 1558–1685.* Cambridge University Press: Cambridge.

13 Black D, Morris J, Smith C, Townsend P (1980) *Inequalities in Health: report of a research working group*. DHSS: London.

14 Acheson D, Barker D, Chambers J, Graham H, Marmot M, Whitehead M (1998) *Independent Inquiry into Inequalities in Health Report*. The Stationery Office: London.

15 Anwar M (1998) *Between Cultures*. Routledge: New York.

16 Commission for Racial Equality (1985) *Immigration Control Procedures*. CRE: London.

17 Anwar M (1996) *British Pakistanis*. Pakistan Forum and Birmingham City Council: Birmingham.

18 Anwar M, Ali A (1987) *Overseas Doctors: experience and expectations*. CRE: London.

19 Anwar M (1991) *Race Relations Policies in Britain: Agenda for the 1990s*. Centre for Research in Ethnic Relations: Coventry.

20 Muslim Council of Britain (2007) *Towards Greater Understanding: meeting the needs of Muslim pupils in state schools*. MCB: London.

21 Runnymede Trust (1997) *Islamophobia: a challenge for us all*. Runnymede Trust: London.

22 Anwar M (1998) *Between Cultures*. Routledge: London.

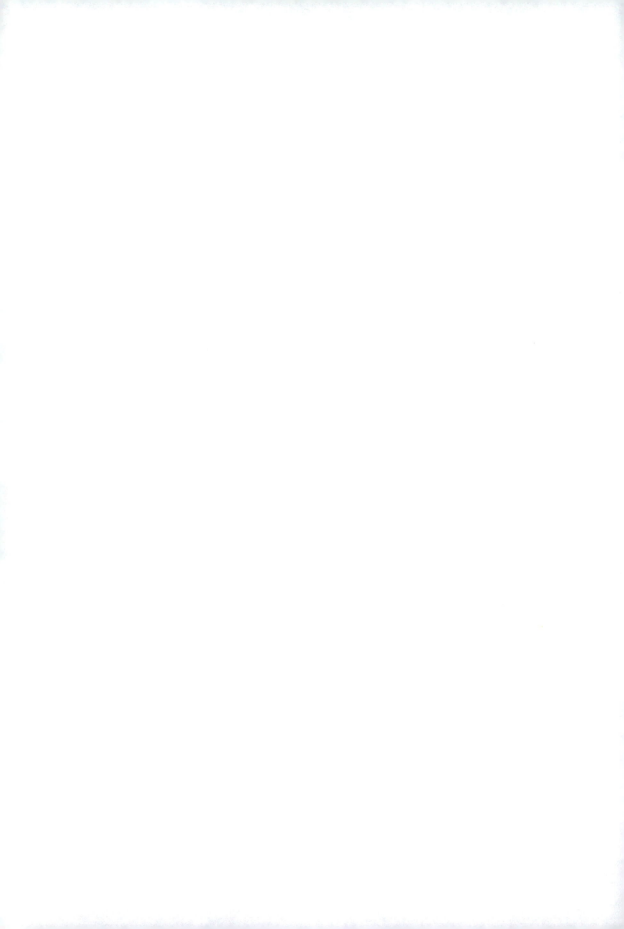

CHAPTER 2

The Muslim grand narrative

☾★ *Tim J Winter*

Islam: a near neighbour

Although Islam has often served as Europe's quintessential 'Other', it is in reality a close sister religion to the Judaism and Christianity which have historically shaped the culture of the West. It shares with them a Middle Eastern origin, and a medieval experience of processes of theological articulation that took place within the context of a shared Greek patrimony. Muslim theology, no less than the religious thought of medieval Christian and Jewish intellectuals such as Aquinas and Maimonides, is a complex and brilliant fusion of the Semitic and the Hellenic spirit: Plato and Moses are the property of Muslims no less than of Christians and Jews. Moreover, Islam is the only non-Christian religion to accord specific recognition to Jesus, the central figure in traditional Western European religion, whom Muslims revere as a healer, a perfect messenger of God (Allah) and as a miracle-working Messiah, although, like Unitarians, Muslims do not accept the doctrine of his divinity.

Despite a superficial strangeness, Islam must hence be classed as a thoroughly Western religion. Its inclusion of Jesus of Nazareth provides one sign of this; but a still more significant connection is supplied by the figure of Abraham. This 'knight of faith' serves for Muslims, as he has for Christians such as Kierkegaard, as the model of a primordial believer, the upholder of a simple monotheism and a pristine moral code. Muhammad, like his forefather Abraham, was cast out by his own people when he opposed their worship of idols and challenged their indifference to the poor; and Islam's holiest site, the Great Sanctuary at Mecca, recalls the Patriarch's desert exile, where Abraham built what the Qur'an describes as the first religious building on earth, the Ka'bah.

Five Pillars of faith

In this sense, the *Hajj*, one of the five cardinal obligations (Table 2.1) that support the spirituality of every observant Muslim, is a rhetorical statement of Islam's understanding of its place in sacred history. The resonances of this spectacular event are powerfully Abrahamic: the seven courses between two Meccan hillocks recall the quest of Hagar for water for the infant Ishmael, a quest which led to the miracle of the Well of Zamzam, which flows to this day. After completing their sevenfold procession around the Ka'bah, the pilgrims pray where Abraham and Ishmael stood during the building of this primordially simple, cubical structure. Later, the culminating ritual takes place at the plain of Arafat, seven miles (11.3 km) from Mecca, where the world's largest multiethnic gathering assembles each year to pray near the Mount of Mercy, revered as the site where the Prophet Muhammad delivered his Farewell Sermon. Standing to petition Allah, pilgrims recall the final resurrection, when Allah, surveying the quality of human hearts, judges the quick and the dead, and decrees their future, beyond time, in heaven or in hell.

TABLE 2.1 The Five Pillars of faith

Shahadah	The testimony of faith.
Salah	The five daily ritual prayers.
Zakat	Annual obligatory alms tax for the poor.
Sawm	Fasting during the month of Ramadan.
Hajj	The annual pilgrimage to Mecca.

The *Hajj* is thus simultaneously the sign of what is familiar and unfamiliar about Islam: it claims Abrahamic ancestry, but with an Ishmaelite voice. Judaism and hence Christianity trace their Abrahamic descent through Isaac, while Islam follows a different covenantal tradition represented in the person of his elder brother Ishmael. The Ishmaelites are marginal to the biblical tradition, but Islam reveres Ishmael as a prophet, whose half-Gentile blood anticipates the destiny of the Ishmaelite covenant to encompass the entire world. Hence Islam's traditional self-image as the only divinely purposed universal religion and as the dispensation designed to bring Abraham to the world. Mirroring this theological hope, the medieval Islamic community stretched across a vast territory from the Pyrenees to Bengal and beyond; and, while recognisably Abrahamic in its beliefs and worship, it acknowledged the specific genius of each of its constituent peoples, who in most cases were not Arabised, but developed their own cultural expressions of the faith, allowing vibrant religious literatures to develop in Persian, Turkish, Hausa, Malay and the hundreds of other vernaculars of the Muslim world. Architecture, from the Great Mosque of Cordova, through the Blue Mosque of Istanbul, to the faience splendours of Isfahan, and still further east, the Taj Mahal, displays this recurrent theme of unity in diversity, of a religious tradition able to accommodate, fertilise and enrich, rather than reduce, the cultures which owe it allegiance. The fact that the Muslim Abraham is seen from so many different angles gives the lie to all stereotypes of Islam as a religious monolith.

The rich diversity of historic Islam, which the *Hajj* symbolises, was further facilitated by the tradition's reluctance to support a hierarchy. Islam has never been, in the conventional sense, 'organised religion'. Its insistence on direct human dealing with a God whose generosity guarantees a gracious response to the prayers and penitence of His creatures eliminates any need for sacraments or for a hierarchy of priests and bishops to administer them. The only authorities are the *Ulema*, literally the 'learned', men and women trained in traditional schools to a level at which they can dispense guidance to others. But these experts possess no automatic authority, and again we find that classical Islam has here embraced an often-bewildering diversity, recognising several distinct theological orientations and at least four canonical traditions of law and worship. Often perceived in the West as univocal, Islamic theology and law have always in reality been richly diverse and, on the many issues which have not been definitively and unambiguously set down in the Muslim scriptures, are showing themselves no less subject to revision in our time than in the past. Issues such as abortion, contraception, genetic engineering, women's roles and many others trigger lively debates among Muslims, disclosing today as never before the absence of an Islamic 'orthodoxy'. Without a church hierarchy to define normality, the tradition slowly evolves by consensus, through discussion of current needs in the light of the scriptures. An absolute uniformity of opinions almost never ensues.

The lack of a hierarchy is evident in another of Islam's 'Five Pillars', the daily worship known as *Salah* (in the Arab world and Africa) and as *Namaz* in Turkey, Iran and the Indian subcontinent. This practice is obligatory for all men and women, if they are sane and adult (adulthood denoting sexual maturity in boys and menarche in girls). Just as the physically frail are excused the *Hajj*, so too those who cannot perform the full movements of the *Salah*, which, in line with Islam's positive view of the body, entails an interaction of physical and spiritual activity, are required to do only what they can accomplish without risk of exacerbating their condition. The healthy must pray in a clean place, usually on a prayer-carpet, facing the Ka'bah, as they recite the Qur'an in Arabic and follow a series of movements which include positions of standing, bowing and prostration. The times appointed for this brief but dignified rite are as follows: *Fajr* (between first light and dawn), *Zuhr* (noon until mid-afternoon), *Asr* (mid-afternoon until sunset), *Maghrib* (just after sunset) and *Isha* (when the sky is completely dark, until midnight, or until the time for *Fajr*).

For those who are able, the *Salah* must be preceded by brief, ritual ablutions known as *wudu* (in Turkish, *abtest*), which entail the washing with clean water of the mouth, nostrils, face, hands and forearms, the wiping of the head and ears, and the washing of the feet. Those too ill to do this carry out the ritual of *tayammum* instead, which simply involves touching a stone or clean dust with both hands, and moving the hands over the face, hands and forearms.[1]

In the lavatory, the practice of *istinja* requires the use of running water to wash the genitals and anus after urination or evacuation. Without this, the *Salah* is not regarded as valid, unless, again, the practice would entail difficulty or danger for a patient. The Prophet Muhammad insisted that those entitled to be excused any such duty carried no blame, and he would grow angry with sick people who, out of misplaced piety, performed ablution rites which might endanger their health.

A further ritual purity practice is *ghusl*. This entails passing clean running water over the entire body (usually today in a shower), and is required after sexual intercourse or ejaculation, and, for women, every month after menstruation has ceased.[2]

The five daily prayers are preferably said in mosques, which, depending on region and custom, may or may not have space for women. In these austere, uncluttered spaces the prayers are led by an *imam*, who may be any male member of the congregation able to recite the Qur'an correctly and to deliver a sermon before the noon congregational prayer each Friday (the *Jum'a* prayer).[3] In some Muslim cultures the *imam* has pastoral responsibilities as well, and may advise on belief and practice, and counsel individuals who seek his help. But although he is a revered figure, his authority is not automatic; neither does he form part of a hierarchy, as typically he is chosen and paid by the local mosque committee, which is answerable only to the congregation. Although *imams* often undertake hospital visits, they have no sacraments to administer, and there are no formal last rites or extreme unction, with the consequence that they are never religiously indispensable. Often patients will prefer to be visited by devout and knowledgeable elders or relations, or by devout members of the local community, whose prayers are regarded as especially reliable.

The duty of *Salah*, then, while formal and often collective, does not locate the believer within a parish or in obedience to a hierarchy. The rite is believed to establish a direct, unmediated connection with the divine presence (the Arabic word *Salah* signifies 'connection'), as symbolised by the turn towards the Ka'bah, and to bring a sense of ease and of burdens lifted. In a parable, the Prophet taught that to pray with sincerity five times in every day resembles washing with the same frequency from a stream running outside one's house. Delayed prayers can lead to anxiety and guilt; prayers performed in serenity trigger a contemplative and relaxed state of mind, a sense of peaceful submission to the will and good providence of Allah, and a state of harmony with the created world, every creature in which, according to the Qur'an, is also adoring Allah in its own way.[4]

The *Salah* links the religious life of the believer to the rolling of the planet beneath his or her feet; while the movements of the moon govern the time of the *Hajj*. The Islamic calendar contains 12 lunar months, with the result that Islamic dates fall some 10 days earlier in each year of the Western calendar. All the festivals hence migrate forward in this way; one of the most conspicuous being *Eid ul-Adha*, which commemorates the end of the *Hajj*. Another festival is *Eid ul-Fitr*, which ends the fasting month of Ramadan.[5]

Although optional fasts are often observed at other times of the year, Ramadan itself is considered one of the Five Pillars of the religion. This key rite, which requires adult, sane and healthy Muslims to abstain from food, drink, tobacco and sexual relations from first light until sunset, forms the subject of a separate chapter in this book (Chapter 8). Religiously it is understood as a means of detaching oneself from worldly, material cravings, thus allowing the spiritual seeker to focus on Allah without distraction. On the moral plane, it is believed to help the rich to empathise with the sufferings of the hungry.

A further technique for achieving spiritual detachment is the practice of *Zakat*. This Arabic word means both 'purification' and 'growth', and refers specifically to the duty to donate one fortieth of one's wealth in charity each year. In the Muslim understanding, wealth is a loan from Allah, and is to be gratefully celebrated by allocating alms for the poor, thereby 'purifying' the remainder and bringing spiritual growth through the practice of renunciation. In addition to the 'Pillar' which is the *Zakat*, the Prophet encouraged his followers to practise alms-giving of a less formal kind, which in the West often takes the form of remittances to needy relations in countries of origin, or of donations to the numerous Muslim charities or to mosques.

The practices of *Salah*, *Hajj*, *Zakat* and the Ramadan fast are simultaneously the expression and strengthening of the core of Muslim theology, which is like a thumb to its four fingers. This is articulated by the *Shahada*, the 'Testimony of Faith', which runs: 'There is no deity but Allah; and Muhammad is Allah's messenger.' This simple creed locates the believer within a world of meaning and identity, the divinely gifted response which is affirmed in the forms of worship, fasting, pilgrimage and charity. It is constantly on the lips of the devout: whispered into the ear of a newborn infant or a dying parent, it frames and defines the believer's experience.

In this way, the Five Pillars of Islam lay down the warp and woof of the Muslim life. The *Shahada* is intended to be a constant presence; the day is punctuated by the five prayers, and the week by the Friday congregational prayer, while the *Zakat* and the Ramadan fast occur once a year, with the *Hajj* coming once in a lifetime. Linking the believer to the movements of the earth, the sun and the moon, these ancient monotheistic rites, practised without alteration since the time of the Prophet, are believed to work a spiritual alchemy on the soul of the Muslim by providing a constant reminder of the beauty and truth which underlie and give meaning to the visible world.

The human condition

The connection with nature, which forms so fundamental a theme of the religion, has a theological basis rooted in the Muslim understanding of the human condition. The Qur'anic account of the Fall differs from the biblical version in allowing Adam a full repentance, thus wiping out the stain of original sin.[6] In Muslim teaching, children are born without sin, so that tendencies to selfishness and vice result from nurture, rather than nature. Heaven and not Hell is the natural destination of humanity even after the Fall; this belief in Allah's generosity is strengthened further by the Prophet's teaching that a good deed is rewarded tenfold. Good intentions, even if not put into practice, are still rewarded by Allah, while bad intentions are not punished if they are never actualised.

Human intelligence is valorised, and the Prophet's dictum that 'the noblest thing Allah has created is the intellect'[7] lies at the root of the Islamic prohibition of alcohol and other narcotics (*see* Chapter 4). Because the body is affirmed as a positive creation of Allah, extreme forms of asceticism and mortification are alien to Muslim piety, as are tattooing and some forms of cosmetic surgery.[8] Sexuality is valued, and the Muslim scriptures confirm that the sex act with one's spouse brings a rich reward from Allah, while celibacy is frowned upon. However, Islam maintains strict standards of sexual morality, forbidding sexual relations with any person to whom one is not married. The seclusion of a man and woman together is regarded as a sign of low standards, as is the unnecessary exposure of the body. Hence women and men are encouraged to dress in a dignified way that often seems at odds with Western norms.[9] In particular, women traditionally cover their bodies when outside their family context, showing only the face, hands and feet. Such traditions, indifference to which can cause considerable embarrassment and discomfort, reflect not only the religion's understanding of public morality and decency but also its theological valorising of the human body, seen as a manifestation of the sacred which must be unveiled only in the most reverent and private context (*see* Chapter 5).[10,11]

Islam's view of humanity may thus be described as upbeat. The Prophet himself 'loved optimism', we are told, and, in the tradition's memory, 'smiled more than any other man'. Without a doctrine of original sin, and with an affirmative attitude to the mind and the body, Muslim cultures have historically favoured a relaxed and genial lifestyle. Medieval castles in England were draughty and austere affairs, while contemporary Muslim palaces, of which the Alhambra in Granada is only the best-known example, were dedicated to the arts of refined and comfortable living. The fall of the Roman Empire prompted the closure of the public baths across Europe; the rise of Islam elevated the public bath (the *hammam*) into a major social institution. Even today, in countries from Morocco to Turkey to the Indian subcontinent, complex massage and grooming practices in the often-splendid surroundings of the *hammam* indicate one way in which Muslims enjoy a religious ethos that combines both hygiene and relaxation.

The way of Muhammad

The spectacular diversity of Muslim cultures has as one point of unity the figure of Abraham, but the practical model and exemplar is always his Ishmaelite descendant, Muhammad.[12] The Prophet of Islam died in the year 632, but as the millions who annually visit his tomb in Madina demonstrate, he remains the role model for Islamic piety and holiness. The Prophet was, quite possibly, the most influential man in history,[13] and although he remains insufficiently known in the West, for Muslims he is revered as a constant inspirational presence. While any idea of his divinity is vigorously resisted, as he called himself 'nothing but Allah's slave', veneration of the Prophet is central to the piety of traditional Muslim cultures and supplies one of the key spiritual energies of the religion.[14] The biblical prohibition on graven images is maintained in Islam, but litanies and poetry, typically of a joyful temper, exist in every Muslim language to describe and sing the Prophet's praises. He is viewed as a hero who suffered persecution and violence from his Meccan contemporaries, and who then, following his migration to Madina in 622, adopted a 'liberation theology' that challenged the tribal structures of Arabia in order to establish a model state in which tribal differences were abolished. Popular themes in devotional literature about the Prophet include his poverty: he lived in a windowless house with a piece of sackcloth for a door and refused to sleep at night until he had given to the poor any food or money which remained in his house. Other themes are his habit of visiting the sick (a particularly meritorious practice in Islam, as those with experience of overcrowded Muslim bedsides will know), his lack of affectation (he often walked barefoot or bareheaded, he swept his house and patched his own clothes), his refusal ever to accept *Zakat* money for himself, and his patience with the often overbearing and crude desert nomads. The reception of the Qur'an, which, as Allah's literal speech conveyed by the Angel Gabriel is regarded as a text so holy that many Muslims will not permit outsiders even to touch it, is considered one of his supreme merits.

A medieval devotional portrait of Muhammad – Allah's final emissary

He maintained friendly and loyal ties with his relatives, but without preferring them to anyone who was superior to them. He never snubbed anyone. He accepted the excuse of anyone who made an excuse. He would joke, but would never say anything that was not true. He would laugh, but not uproariously. He would watch permissible games and sports, and would not criticise them. He ran races with his wives. Voices would be raised around him, and he would be patient. He kept a sheep, from which he would draw milk for his family. He would walk among the fields of his companions. He never despised any pauper for his poverty or illness; neither did he hold any king in awe simply because he was a king. He would call rich and poor to Allah, without distinction.

– Abu Hamid al-Ghazali1[15]

Love for the Prophet is hence central in the Muslim affective range. Allah is held in awe and respect; the Prophet is loved. Thus committed Muslims never utter or hear his name without repeating the words, 'Allah bless him and send him peace!' (*salla'Llahu alayhi wa-sallam*). This love in turn informs and energises a cardinal duty of the faith, which is the faithful emulation of the Prophet's *Sunnah*: his custom, or way of life. The Muslim *imitatio* of the Prophet can appear odd to outsiders, and only becomes coherent in the light of the emotion of love and reverence in which the 'Best of Creation' is held. Pious Muslims regard his human and spiritual perfection as a model to be emulated in all circumstances. He ate sitting on a rug on the floor, using his right hand, after invoking Allah; many traditional Muslims do likewise. The interior of a fully traditional Muslim home recalls the simplicity of the Prophet's life: the absence of furniture is believed to engender an atmosphere of uncluttered serenity. To sit on the floor, Muslims believe, in the mosque or at home, serves to reduce the emotional distance between fellow human beings.

Love for the Prophet also animates more formal aspects of Muslim tradition such as dietary rules. Pork is forbidden, as is the flesh of animals or birds whose lives have been taken by idolaters or atheists. Fish is permissible, as is lamb, beef or chicken slaughtered by Muslims in a way which is *halal* (permissible). Most Muslims will eat kosher meat, as this is prepared in a similar way and has been slaughtered by believers in God; many Muslims will also eat meat killed by Christians.

Again following the Prophet's example, there are traditions of effusive greeting involving handshaking and embraces, accompanied by the phrase *Assalamu-Alaikum*: 'Peace be upon you'.

The *Sunnah* is applicable to both sexes, with important differentiation; although the debate over women's rights and roles is sharp in modern Islam, with believers defending a wide spectrum of opinions, Muslims are anxious to point to the evidence for Islam's high esteem for women.[16,17] Because Allah is ungendered, there is no cosmic prioritising of the male principle. The Five Pillars are incumbent upon both sexes, and salvation is open to men and women alike. In many Muslim societies the oppression of women is frequent, as it is in many other traditional cultures (such as some Christian cultures of Latin America or certain Hindu environments), but Muslims insist that such abuses are the product of un-Islamic cultural values that have survived an Islamisation process that has seldom been much more than partial. For this reason women have often been at the forefront of calls to bring to the modern Muslim world forms of Islamic government, however variously this is understood.

The major Islamic denominations recognise the decisive authority of the Prophet's *Sunnah*. Ninety per cent of the world's Muslims (and an even higher percentage in the West) are *Sunnis*, who subscribe to the version of Islam outlined in this chapter. The great majority of the remainder are *Shi'is* (collectively known as *Shi'a*), who were distinguished from the mainstream community after the Prophet's death on the basis of their conviction that his descendants alone should be the successors to his temporal authority. The practical and doctrinal differences between *Sunnis* and *Shi'is* are relatively slight, perhaps the most conspicuous being the *Shi'a* practice of combining prayers so as to pray on only three occasions in each day, and of breaking the fast at least half an hour after sunset.

Sunnis and *Shi'is* share one view and experience of Islam, which is that it represents all imaginable human compassion and dignity. Western images, fed by a mass media preoccupied with extremist minorities and indifferent to mainstream piety, are unrecognisable and often deeply offensive to traditional believers, for whom Islam is nothing less than a synonym for goodness. Stripped of cultural encrustation or associations with political extremism, it is a religion which is not only easily understood, given the simplicity of its doctrine and the optimism of its world-view, but is also easily respected for the standards which it introduces to the often confused moral landscape of contemporary Western societies.

Summary

- ⇢ Although frequently perceived as an 'outsider', Islam is in fact a close sister religion to Judaism and Christianity. Born of the same ancient Semitic soil, Islam regards itself as nothing other than a continuation and culmination of the pristine message of the biblical prophets.
- ⇢ Core aspects of the Muslim faith, namely the insistence on monotheism, a regard for the sacred in all walks of life and belief in a final accountability, are very intimately linked to the Judeo-Christian narrative, which has traditionally shaped the culture of the West.
- ⇢ Many of the most evident aspects of Muslim culture, such as race, dress customs, cookery and language, are functions not of the religion proper, but of the specifics of regional culture in the countries of origin. Islam continues to respect and value such diversity, so long as it does not transgress the boundaries of Sacred Law.
- ⇢ The end to primary immigration of Muslims will lead to an inexorable increase in the percentage of Western-born Muslims. Though these second- and third-generation Western Muslims are discarding aspects of regional culture, core values of the faith remain strong, thereby allowing the strong doctrinal and moral affinity between Islam and more traditional aspects of European religion and culture to become more widely recognised.
- ⇢ For the majority of Muslims, Islam is nothing less than a synonym for goodness.

References

1 Keller NHM (1995) *The Reliance of the Traveller*, pp. 60–92. Amana: Maryland.
2 Ibid., pp. 93–5.
3 Children, the sick and the frail elderly are not required to attend any mosque service.
4 Sheikh A (1997) Quiet room is needed in hospitals for prayer and reflection. *BMJ*. **315**: 1625.

5 Ahsan MM (1985) *Muslim Festivals*. Wayland: Hove.

6 Anawati MM (1958) Islam and the immaculate conception. In: D O'Connor (ed) *The Dogma of the Immaculate Conception*. University of Notre Dame Press: Notre Dame.

7 al-Munajjid SA (1987) *Al-'Aql*, p. 12. Dar Nasr: Beirut.

8 Rispler-Chaim V (1993) *Islamic Medical Ethics in the Twentieth Century*. Brill: Leiden.

9 Naficy H (1999) Veiled visions, powerful presences. In: R Issa, R Whitaker (eds) *Life and Art: the new Iranian cinema*. National Film Theatre: London.

10 Bouhdhiba A (1985) *Sexuality in Islam*. Routledge: London.

11 Musallam B (1983) *Sex and Society in Islam*. Cambridge University Press: Cambridge.

12 Lings M (1993) *Muhammad: his life based on the earliest sources*. George Allen and Unwin: London.

13 If we divide the credit for the foundation of Christianity between Christ and St Paul, this is a readily defensible position.

14 Schimmel A (1985) *And Muhammad is His Messenger: the veneration of the Prophet in Islamic piety*. University of North Carolina Press: Chapel Hill.

15 al-Ghazali AH (1927) *Ihya' 'Ulum al-Din* (The revival of the religious sciences), vol II, pp. 319–20. al-Halabi: Cairo.

16 Badawi L (1994) Islam. In: J Holm, J Bowker (eds) *Women in Religion*. Pinter: London.

17 Murata S (1992) *The Tao of Islam: a sourcebook on gender relationships in Islamic thought*. State University of New York Press: Albany.

CHAPTER 3

Health and disease: an Islamic framework

(★ *Abdul Aziz Ahmed*

An individual's understanding of concepts such as 'health' and 'disease' arise from a complex interaction between personal experiences and a range of cultural factors that may include, among other things, language, family values and norms, and religion.[1] The relative importance of each of these factors in determining one's outlook may vary quite substantially between cultures, and, in pluralist societies such as those that now characterise many parts of the Western world, from one subculture to another. In those communities that retain a sense of the sacred, the influence of religion on shaping the individual and communal view is often quite considerable.[2] My experience of studying, teaching and living with disparate Muslim communities, in four different continents, suggests that this is certainly true with respect to Muslims. An appreciation of religious ethic surrounding health and disease may therefore aid professionals in the challenging role of delivering care in a manner that is appropriate and culturally sensitive.[3] This chapter delineates and explores the nature of health and ill health from within the Islamic world-view. An etymological approach is adopted, drawing on Qur'anic lexicons and Arabic commentaries on classical Islamic texts, for linguistic competence and religious understanding are regarded as inseparable within classical Muslim thought.

Health, disease and the human heart

There is in the body a piece of flesh, and if it is good the entire body is good. However, if it is diseased, the entire body is diseased; and know, it is the heart.

– Prophet Muhammad [4]

Man's essence

Man – Allah's masterpiece creation – is fundamentally different from all other beings. The most important distinction is that he has both an external and internal reality. His external being, his corpus, is that which he shares with the rest of creation. The central point of his inwardness, the domain of the spirit and soul, is the *qalb*, or the human heart. The human stands distinct and indeed elevated above all else in creation, whether in the animal or angelic realm, on account of this inward dimension, for this is his essence – the isthmus between the temporal and eternal worlds. Ultimately then, all humans will be judged according to the 'health' of this inner reality, for as the Prophet constantly reminded the women and men of faith, 'Allah does not look to your bodies, nor your forms, but rather He looks to your hearts.'

The second chapter, *The Muslim grand narrative*, described how Man's separation from the Divine, following Adam's Fall, is temporary – his intended destiny is one of return. Born healthy, in a primordial pure state (*al-fitra*), so long as he preserves and maintains this condition he can be assured that his lot in the eternal life hereafter will be one of bliss, satisfaction, and a deep and lasting peace.

Qalb, an Arabic term, refers to 'the essence and most inner aspect of a thing', differentiating and demarcating it from all else. The *qalb* of a palm tree, for example, is the seed of its fruit. Without a seed the date could not and would not have existed. If a tree produces no seed, it is, in the desert Arab's view, useless, but through its seeds it is eternal. The 'healthy heart' that is mentioned in the Prophetic tradition cited above is thus far more than a strong and efficient coronary organ.

The states of the heart

And let me not be in disgrace on the Day when men will be raised up; the Day when neither wealth nor sons will avail, but only he will prosper that brings to Allah a sound heart.

– Qur'an [5]

And in their hearts is a disease.

– Qur'an[6]

The verb from which the word *qalb* is derived also means 'to turn' (*yan qalibo*). The heart can turn in many directions. In whichever direction it turns the body will follow, for as al-Ghazali (d. 1111) – the celebrated medieval theologian and logician – remarked of the heart, 'it is the king who is obediently followed by the other limbs; if the king is upright and good then his servants will be likewise'.[7]

In Arabic, one who is sound and healthy is said to be *salim*. Classical Arabic dictionaries define *salim* as 'the one who has been stung or bitten by a snake'.[8] In pre-Islamic Arabia, the snakebite was considered to be a good omen, indicating future well-being. With the arrival of Islam the meaning of *salim* evolved. Muslims began to see a healthy state, or the state of being *salim*, as one in which a person can see the will of Allah even in times of adversity and tribulation – being bitten by a desert snake was but one example of such an affliction.

The *salim* will therefore not see illness as a punishment, but rather as a 'test' from Allah; these tests that we experience at many junctures throughout life afford the opportunity to deal with many of the ills of the heart (Table 3.1) – the diseases of material attachment and the associated tendency to forget Allah, for example. According to an oft-repeated tradition, sickness and tribulation bring an opportunity to earn reward through patience and steadfastness and are a cause for the cleansing of one's sins. The Prophet said: 'No Muslim will be afflicted by hardship or illness, or anxiety or worry, or harm or sadness, even the pricking of a thorn, except that, by it, Allah will cover up some of his sins'.[9] It has been argued by some Muslim scholars that the greater the illness, the greater is the reward. While the Prophet lay dying with fever, one of his companions suggested that his pain and fever was twice that of others. When he enquired whether this indicated that he would receive a double reward, the Prophet responded in the affirmative, adding: 'A Muslim is not afflicted with illness, or the like, other than (through this experience) Allah sheds from him his mistakes, just like a tree sheds its leaves.'[10]

TABLE 3.1   The states of the heart

THE HEALTHY HEART	THE DISEASED HEART
Belief in Allah	Disbelief in Allah
Sincerity of purpose	Hypocrisy
Humility	Arrogance
Hope in Allah's good Providence	Despairing of Allah's mercy
Contentment	Dissatisfaction
Regard for Sacred Law	Disdain for Sacred Law
Divine Love	Material and temporal love

Muslim literature is rich with accounts of the companions of the Prophet, who would often worry, thinking Allah had forsaken them if they went for extended periods without being afflicted or, from their perspective, blessed through illness. This does not, however, mean that they actively sought situations where physical ailments were likely, or that they failed to seek a cure when problems occurred. On the contrary, based on the advice and encouragement of the Prophet, from the earliest times Muslims have been committed to and engaged in medicinal practice (*see below*).

In Semitic languages, words are generally derived from a three-lettered root term. A number of related words stem from this same root, and an appreciation of these derivatives helps in developing a fuller understanding of the concept being considered. *Salim* then is derived from the root S-L-M; other derivatives of this term include *salama* (safety), *salaam* (the Muslim greeting of peace), *Islam* (the way of peace) and *Muslim* (one who has voluntarily surrendered his will to the Divine will, and so is in a state of peace). A *qalb salim*, or healthy heart, when considered in its fullest sense, is an organ that is whole, sound, content and at peace, directing the rest of the body in the pursuit of good, where good is defined as following of Sacred Law. Since this is the path that leads back to the Ancestral Home there can be no higher good. Similar meanings can be found in other sacred cultures – healing and holiness stem from the same root term for example, both words suggesting a sense of wholeness, a theme that dominated early and medieval Christian notions of health.[11]

An Arab maxim teaches that to understand a particular notion one must understand its antithesis. If a healthy heart leads towards eternity, the diseased heart (*qalb marid*) is preoccupied with the temporal, content in self-gratification, self-indulgence and a disregard for Sacred Law. One with a diseased heart will thus neither be able to contextualise illness nor know how to conduct himself or herself in such a situation. Despair, discontentment and dissatisfaction with Allah's plan characterises an unsound heart in such situations. Many of the psychological problems that plague today's world, stress, anxiety and depression to mention but a few, reflect the improvised condition of modern man.[12] In his arrogance he fails to recognise the very essence of being, and is as a result deprived of any inward sustenance.

Hope and fear – qualities of a sound heart

A young man lay dying at the time of the Prophet Muhammad. 'How are you?' enquired the Prophet. 'Hoping in my Lord, but fearful on account of my sins' came the reply. The Prophet then declared: 'Never do these two emotions unite in the heart of a Muslim, in such a situation as this, but that Allah gives him what he hopes for, and gives him safekeeping from that which he fears'.[13]

Healing the heart

The Qur'an makes little mention of physical illness, its primary focus being attending to the state of the heart. Through a combination of encouragement, enticement, warning and exhortation it seeks to remind (*dhikr*) the human heart, an organ that is liable to frequently forget its true purpose, of the transience of the life of this world and the reward that awaits those who remain steadfast and pure. It is for this reason that the Qur'an – Allah's final revelation – chooses to describe itself as *As-Shifa*, or 'a healing', asserting categorically that 'it is only in the mention of Allah that hearts find rest'.[14]

The physical state

> Allah did not send down a sickness except that He sent down its cure.
>
> – *Prophet Muhammad*[15]

The rights of the body

Sacred Law articulates certain rights to the body, above all being the right that it is accorded respect, whether in life or death, for by definition man is its temporary custodian. The body needs to be maintained and attended to and it is for this very reason that much of Sacred Law exists, with its insistence on matters of cleanliness and personal hygiene, wholesome food and drink (*halal*), and providing the body with the due amounts of exercise and rest. The concept of 'balance' is central to the Qur'anic message, for just as the cosmos is in balance, so must be its principal inhabitant.

The development of healthcare

'There is a cure for every malady save one – that of old age'[16] said the noble Prophet in a famous tradition, placing a personal responsibility on the one with an ailment to seek its remedy. For this, rather than use incantations or sorcery, as was common in pre-Islamic Arabia, the believers were encouraged to seek the services of one trained in the appropriate sciences, while nonetheless being aware that cure ultimately resides in the hands of *As-Shafi*, 'The Supreme Healer'.[17]

Traditionally this call has been heeded with seriousness, and it is interesting to note that one of the first sciences to flourish in the lands won over to Islam was that of medicine. Notions of an imbalance in the humours, as was the prevalent belief in Antiquity, resonated with the views of many within the early Muslim communities, acting as a catalyst for the so-called 'age of translations'. This was by anyone's accounts a most remarkable episode in the history of medicine, for while much of Europe had plundered into 'The Dark Ages', Christian and Muslim scholars, under official state patronage, were busy translating, commenting on and critiquing Greek, and also Persian and Indian, medical scholarship, seeking improved understanding, and ultimately cure, for conditions for which effective remedies were lacking. Interest in medicinal practice has always been central to Muslim piety, for there are literally scores of prophetic traditions placing great esteem on helping and aiding one's fellow man in his hour of need.

With access to the learning that had accrued over centuries in many of the most important traditions of the time, Muslim scholarship quickly turned its attention to the synthesis and dissemination of this body of teaching. The towering figures of the Persian philosopher-physicians Muhammad ibn-Zakariya al-Rhazi (d. 925) and Abu Ali al-Husayn ibn Abdullah ibn Sina (d. 1037), known to the West as Rhazes and Avicenna respectively, represent the pinnacle of this synthesis phase, with their compendia dominating medical curricula in the Muslim and Christian worlds for well over five centuries. The Spanish-born Abul-Qasim al-Zahrawi (d. 1013) and Ahmad ibn Muhammad ibn Rushd (d. 1198), Latinized as Albucasis and Averroes respectively, indicate the breadth and depth of the learning and dissemination culture that the Qur'an, with its repeated emphasis on learning and teaching, fostered.[18]

Improvements in clinical care were of paramount importance, and much important advancement was made to existing practice. These included the first network of regular and mobile hospitals (*bimaristan*) seeking to offer medical care free of charge, irrespective of gender, race or religious affiliation, and the first centres devoted to the humane care of the insane (*maristan*). Considerable advancements were made in the field of medical ethics (*see* Chapter 4), the most notable contributions coming from the pen of one Ishaq ibn Ali al-Rahawi who, during the second half of the 9th century, laid the foundations for *Adab al-Tabib* (The Ethics of the Physician), reminding physicians that they were charged with maintaining both body and soul. Medical education and registration were other fields that benefited from Muslim contributions, with the concept of re-accreditation of physicians gaining importance for the first time in 10th-century Baghdad.[18,19]

The potted and sketchy history of Muslim contributions to medicine here presented is in no way meant to be comprehensive, but rather to reflect the importance attached to medicine from the earliest of times. The oft-repeated myth that Muslims' sole contribution to medicine (and the sciences) was the preservation of Hellenistic learning owes more to the imperialistic vision that characterised post-Enlightenment Europe than to any objective reading of history. This interest continues, as evidenced by the desire of many a Muslim parent that their children enter the healing profession, and in view of the Qur'anic reminder – 'That whosoever saves a human life, it is as if they have saved the whole of humankind'[20] – that such sentiments are expressed should perhaps come as no great surprise.

Children's ode in honour of Avicenna – 'Prince of Physicians'

Many may be clever, but few are truly wise
For wisdom shows you things that are hidden from men's eyes
Avicenna was given wisdom before he came of age
And proved while still a beardless youth that he was already a great sage.

Exporting the Qur'anic framework

Arabic – the language of the Qur'an – is the source *par excellence* through which Muslim culture traces its roots. As non-Arab nations embraced the Islamic vision, they adopted many Arabic terms for key concepts. The degree to which this occurred varied from region to region. Northwest Africa, for example, became almost completely Arabised, while other regions, such as Southeast Asia, only assimilated religious terms. The impact of Qur'anic Arabic in these latter regions should not, however, be underestimated because although only a few hundred terms may have been adopted, many of these have assumed positions of pivotal importance in defining important concepts in these communities. The word *afiya*, for example, which denotes a sense of wholeness and totality, is used in modern Swahili for health; similarly, *dawa*, signifying a means to achieve cure, is currently used in Urdu for medication. With the transfer of these Qur'anic terms came a shift in, or refinement of, these concepts. Perhaps most noteworthy of all is that the greeting of peace – *Assalamu-Alaikum* (a derivative of *salim*) – is in universal use among Muslims, be they in majority or minority communities. These few examples illustrate the extent to which such Qur'anic terms have permeated the language and culture of non-Arab Muslim nations.

Where worlds meet

No, no, I disagree!

'Depression is very common in the Muslim community, and our attempts at treating it effectively are hampered by the stigma attached to the diagnosis,' opined a Muslim psychiatrist.

'It's not right to consider depression as a physical illness – depression reflects a lack of faith,' retorted someone from the floor.

Exasperated, the psychiatrist tried again: 'You see; this is just what I mean!'

There then followed a long, and at times, heated discussion on Islamic perspectives on health and disease. After considerable discussion and debate, and with no clear conclusions drawn, the Chairman tactfully steered the discussion on to a less contentious issue.

– Muslim Health Conference, London

Familiar to anthropologists is the phenomenon of acculturation – the process through which a minority group will incorporate some of the cultural attributes of the larger society. Being confronted with a post-Enlightenment Western tradition that has all but neglected the inner reality, and for whom the heart is considered no more than a biological pump, has for many Muslims caused considerable dissonance with the traditional view of understanding health and disease. Being caught between contrasting and at times conflicting world-views has resulted in confusion among some Western Muslims regarding their personal interpretations of health and disease.

A focus on physical health, and attempts at understanding disease states of the heart such as anger, discontentment and caprice in biological terms, or perhaps even more seriously as *normal* human emotions, leaves many in a state of inner turmoil. The 'aches and pains' and 'heartache' so common among Muslims possibly represents an attempt to articulate this turmoil in a form that may be understood by clinicians. Frequent recourse to the diagnostic dumping ground of 'difficult' or 'heart-sink' indicates the miserable failure of many such attempts, exemplifying the difficulty of communicating across and between paradigms. The mass search for 'alternative' or 'complementary' cures now under way throughout the Western world suggests that it is not only Muslims that are being left short by biomedicine.[21] By focusing on the external reality, the corpus, modern medicine is failing to reach its true potential.

Summary

- An individual's understanding of notions of health and disease arise from a complex interplay between personal experience and cultural factors such as language and religion.
- For communities with a sacred tradition the influence of religious ethic in shaping this outlook is likely to be strong.
- Traditional Islamic teaching considers disease states of two kinds: spiritual and physical. Spiritual ill health is the more serious since the Prophet taught: 'Allah does not look to your bodies nor your forms, but rather He looks to your hearts.'
- Islamic teaching obliges Muslims to seek cures for both spiritual and physical disease. The former are usually sought from those trained in understanding inner realities, i.e. teachers of religion, while the latter are sought from those trained in the physical sciences – many in the Muslim world are trained in both of these disciplines. Cure, however, comes solely from Allah and these individuals and institutions are simply Allah's instruments for effecting cure.
- The Muslim community in many Western societies is currently in an acculturation phase with respect to its understanding of health and disease.

References

1 Helman CG (2001) *Culture, Health and Illness.* Arnold: London.
2 Rahman F (1998) *Health and Medicine in the Islamic Tradition.* ABC: Chicago.
3 Lee L (1997) *Breaking Barriers: towards culturally competent general practice.* RCGP: London.
4 Khan MM (1990) *Sahih al-Bukhari.* Dar Al-arabia: Beirut.
5 Ali YA (1938) *The Meaning of the Glorious Quran;* **26**: 87–89 (trans modified). Dar al-Kitab: Cairo.
6 Ali YA (1938) *The Meaning of the Glorious Quran;* **2**: 10 (trans modified). Dar al-Kitab: Cairo.
7 al-Ghazali AH (1923) *Minhaj al-abideen.* Maktaba Isha'at al-Islam: Delhi.
8 ibn Daqiq al-'Eid (1983) *Sharh al-Arabain.* Dar al-Kutub al-'ilmiya: Beirut.
9 Khan MM (1980) *Sahih al-Bukhari;* **vii**: 371–72. Dar al-Arabia: Beirut.
10 Sabiq AS (1989) *Fiqh us-sunnah;* **iv**: 1. ATP: Indianapolis.
11 Porter R (1997) *The Greatest Benefit to Mankind,* p. 84. Harper Collins: London.
12 Nasr SH (1997) *The Spiritual Crisis in Modern Man.* ABC: Chicago.
13 Sahih al-Tirmidhi (1996) In: SN Shah (ed) *The Alim for Windows.* ISL Software Corporation.
14 Ali YA (1938) *The Meaning of the Glorious Quran;* **13**: 28 (trans modified). Dar al-Kitab: Cairo.
15 Khan MM (1980) *Sahih al-Bukhari;* **vii**: 395. Dar al-Arabia: Beirut.
16 Johnstone P (1998) *Ibn Qayyim al-Jawziyya Medicine of the Prophet,* p. 10. Islamic Texts Society: Cambridge.
17 Al-Halveti TB (1985) *The Most Beautiful Names.* Threshold: Vermont.
18 Rahman F (1989) Islam and health/medicine: a historical perspective. In: LE Sullivan (ed) *Healing and Restoring: health and medicine in the world's religious traditions,* pp. 149–72. Macmillan: New York.
19 Surty MI (1996) *Muslims' Contribution to the Development of Hospitals.* Qur'anic Arabic Foundation: Birmingham.
20 Ali YA (1938) *The Meaning of the Glorious Quran;* **5**: 32 (trans modified). Dar al-Kitab: Cairo.
21 Eisenberg DM, Kessler RC, Foster C, Norlock FE, Calkins DR, Delbanco TL (1993) Unconventional medicine in the United States: prevalence, costs, and patterns of use. *NEJM;* **328**: 246–52.

CHAPTER 4

Principles of Islamic bioethics

(★ *Hamza Yusuf Hanson*

Introduction

To encounter Islam is to encounter a comprehensive tradition that encompasses all areas of the human condition. This includes medical treatment. Islam has a rich medical history, and has encouraged the pursuit of medical science. As the Prophet Muhammad said, 'Seek medical treatment, O servants of God, for surely medical treatment is part of God's Providence.'[1]

Islam is deeply concerned with living according to God's will, and in consequence developed a comprehensive sacred legal system by which to discern the best course of action in any circumstance. For it must be understood that Islam is both a faith and a legal system. Indeed, the two are inseparable – the legal system acting as the practical guide to living according to faith. This faith bases itself firmly on the received revelation of the Qur'an and the prophetic traditions of Muhammad, and the legal system functions as an apparatus for deciding and guiding the appropriateness of actions based upon these traditions and revelations. In other words, the legal system is a system of ethics. And as all action springs from the human body, it is only natural for Islam to be interested in the practice of medicine.

Islam and medicine

As medical practice developed under the sphere of Islam, legal jurists became more and more interested in analysing the practices of medicine in reference to tradition and revelation. Eventually, many wanted to place medical practice within the confines of Sacred Law. Yet others disagreed. The 14th century scholar Ibn Khaldun says:

> The medicine mentioned in religious tradition is of the Bedouin type. It is in no way part of the divine revelation. Such medical matters were merely part of Arab custom and happened to be mentioned in connection with the circumstances of the Prophet, like other things that were customary in his generation. They were not mentioned in order to imply that that particular way of practicing medicine is stipulated by religious law. Muhammad was sent to teach us the religious law. He was not sent to teach us medicine or any other ordinary matter.[2]

However, some Muslims still shun modern medical practices because they believe that only the primitive medical methods and practices during the time of Muhammad are sanctioned by God. But this has never been more than a minority position. Most Muslims have always remained open to improvements in medical science, and Islam (as opposed to the Christian West) has never been adverse or opposed to science.

Originally, the medical practices of Arabia at the time of the Prophet Muhammad were very primitive. Yet as Islam spread out across the world, Muslims quickly acquired new knowledge and came to incorporate the sophisticated medical practices of Persia, India and the Byzantine.

To this knowledge they added their own understandings. Taking from the Qur'an and the prophetic traditions, a medical school known as *Tibb an-Nabawi* or 'Prophetic Medicine' sprung up. This school believed that both the Qur'an and the prophetic tradition give sound medical principles regarding the maintenance and restoration of health. One such example is the saying of Muhammad, 'Fast and restore your health.'[3] Moreover, according to Ibn Qayyim al-Jauzia's famous treatise on Prophetic Medicine, you can ascertain from the Qur'an and the prophetic traditions that medical science consists of three basic principles: preserving good health, avoiding what harms one's body, and ridding the body of toxins.[4]

In addition, Islamic medicine deals with an area of study often neglected by other medical sciences: spiritual diseases. Spiritual diseases include such conditions as envy, avarice, anxiety, and obsessive/compulsive disorders. These diseases are seen as psychopathological, and according to Islamic medicine are to be treated and diagnosed just as any other ailment or condition.

When it comes to deciding on a medical treatment, the final decision belongs to the individual. While the Qur'an counsels to 'Ask the people of knowledge if you do not know,' the final choice on whether a course of treatment is acceptable to Islamic ethics remains with the individual. The reason for this is simple: the scholars often disagree. Moreover, it is recognised that in absence of any clear statement in either the Qur'an or prophetic traditions, a scholar's opinion is still a human attempt to discern the will of God – and as such, does not have the force of law. The Prophet Muhammad even encouraged these disagreements. As he says, 'Differences of opinion among my community is from God's Mercy.'

Five legal rulings

In helping to determine the ethicality of any action, Islam provides an elegant legal methodology. To begin with, every action is grouped under one of five legal rulings: obligatory (*fard*), recommended (*mandub*), permitted (*mubah*), discouraged (*makruh*), and prohibited (*haram*). At the basic level, every action is considered permissible unless a clear proof establishing its prohibition is provided. This proof would take the form of an explicit textual prohibition, or, through analogical reasoning, be determined impermissible based on a similarity to some other textually prohibited action. One such example of a prohibited action is the consumption of alcohol. But, overall, unless specifically ruled prohibited, any medical treatment is considered permissible.

Two principles, three states and six universals

Islamic legal methodology is considered rational and not arbitrary. Therefore, through understanding a few principles, categories and states, any person can come to a reasonable understanding of a legal ruling. For example, the entire Islamic legal system can arguably be reduced to two principles: 'the accruement of benefit' (*jalb al-maslahah*) and 'the warding off of harm' (*dar' al-mafsadah*). The warding off of harm is always considered to take priority over the accruement of benefit, and in this consideration we have a first basic rational method for determining the ethicality of any action.

Beyond the two principles, every action can be classified under three categorical states. The first category is 'necessary' (*darurat*), and involves any situation that preserves one of the six 'universals': religion, life, sanity, property, lineage, and human dignity. In preservation of these necessary universals, several prohibitions have been enacted. A few of the prohibitions are as follows: the prohibition of religious tolerance to preserve religion, the prohibition of murder to preserve life, the prohibition of intoxicants to preserve sanity, the prohibition of theft to preserve property, the prohibition of adultery to preserve lineage, and the prohibition of slander or calumny to preserve human dignity.

The second categorical state is the 'needed' (*hajiyyat*), and the third is the 'comforting' (*tahsiniyyat*). The needed category includes all matters that help maintain the six universals without hardship. The comforts are those matters which add to the joy and experience of life. As it says in the Qur'an, 'Say: who can prohibit the good things of life that God has brought for His creation to enjoy?'[5]

An Islamic legal ruling that permits what is normally prohibited is often arrived at through the process of determining which category a particular action falls under. Once a category is determined, a ruling could override a prohibition if it means preserving or regaining a more important matter from a category that takes precedence over the category from which the particular prohibition arises. For example, the act of having children is generally placed in the third category of comfort. Therefore, it would not be considered permissible for a woman to have surgery that may be life threatening in order to be able to bear children. The preservation of her life overrides the comfort of having children.[6]

Five golden principles

The methods that jurists use to determine a legal ruling involve many variables and considerations and the above-mentioned principles and categories are just part of a comprehensive methodology. While there are several hundred principles within the four major legal schools in Islam, there are actually five major principles that are seen as the matrixes for all of the others.

The first is, 'all matters are judged based upon the intended outcomes'. In other words, it is generally prohibited to stab someone, but in the case of a surgeon, for example, whose intention is to heal and not to harm, the ruling for his cutting the flesh of the patient differs from a man who stabs another to steal his wealth. While this is a simplified and obvious case, the principle has far-reaching implications in Islamic legal reasoning.

The second is, 'necessity permits the impermissible'. This is a fundamental principle known and understood by most practising Muslims. For instance, Muslims are prohibited from consuming pork and wine. However, when a person is in a life-threatening situation, it becomes permissible – in fact an obligation – to consume either of them if it would prevent loss of life. This would be the case should one be starving, and pork is the only sustenance found, or if someone is choking or dying of thirst and wine is the only substance available. In both cases, the necessity of life preservation outweighs the prohibition of the substance. This ruling is particularly important in matters of medical practice insofar as it has been used by scholars to permit such procedures as organ transplants and blood transfusions.

The third principle is 'hardship engenders facilitation'. This principle is already acted upon considerably in medical practice. Take the use of anaesthetising drugs, for instance. In normal circumstances, these drugs would be prohibited, but because their effects are considered temporary and undergoing certain medical procedures without them results in undue hardship to the patient, scholars have generally permitted their use, including drugs like morphine and similar painkillers.

The fourth principle is 'conditions never become constricting except that relief must be facilitated'. This is similar to the previous principle but has more general application in that it relates to the group as opposed to the individual. Essentially, it holds that when large numbers are affected by conditions, the ruling changes. An example of this is water's purity for devotional practices. Generally, to be purifying for ritual use, water must not be altered in taste, smell or colour. Thus the smell and taste of chlorinated water would normally make it impure for devotional use because they are not part of its natural state, whereas sea water would be acceptable because its salty taste does not affect the ruling of the water, given that it is a characteristic of its natural state. Nonetheless, the majority of scholars have ruled that water chlorinated for hygienic reasons (that is, to guard the health of those using it) overrides the normal ruling.

The fifth principle is 'harm is always removed'. This is a far-reaching principle in medicine. It maintains that the foundation of health is being free from harmful states, and based upon this principle whatever can be done in most cases to remove harm is permissible.

Medication

Drugs, according to Islamic Law, are categorised under three legal and not medical classes: intoxicants (*muskirat*), anaesthetics (*muraqqidat*), and corrupting (*mufsidat*). This classification goes back several hundred years but was clearly explained by Shibadin Al-Qarafi in the 13th century in his authoritative book *Al-Furuuq*, where he categorised them saying,

> There are three types of drugs. [The first is] those that anaesthetise the five senses completely, and we call these muraqqidat. [The next two are] those that do not anaesthetise: the first is intoxicants, which inebriate and cause a feeling of excitement and well-being; these are muskirat. The second [which is corrupting drugs (mufsidat in Arabic)] affects the intellect but does not cause a sense of joy or exhilaration. Hashish is an example of such a corrupting drug. Intoxicants differ from both anaesthetics and corrupting drugs in three ways: 1) there is a specified legal punishment for the use of intoxicants; 2) they are considered impure substances; and 3) a small amount is still prohibited. As for anaesthetics and corrupting drugs, they are pure in substance, there is no specified punishment for their users, and a small amount that does not affect the intellect is permissible.[7]

Generally, Muslim scholars permitted drug use for excruciating pain relief. Muslims are also to generally avoid using medications that have alcohol bases. However, if there are no alternatives and they are deemed necessary or needful as opposed to comforting, then they are permissible. The same is true with pig-based insulin and other medications that have unclean constituents. Bone is also problematic in transplants and grafting, but is permissible if necessary.

Medical malpractice

An important aspect of medical ethics in Islam is the prudent practice required of a physician or any other healthcare worker. While medical malpractice is a modern concept in the West, Muslim jurists considered the physician obliged to provide indemnity for any harm caused by incautious actions. In fact, jurists put limits on the monetary compensation for all organ and limb damage and determined specific amounts for each one as well as loss of life. The habit of paying such indemnities was common during the Prophet Muhammad's lifetime and is thus considered revelation by the jurists. These laws are still binding upon practising Muslims and actually apply to Muslims who might sue non-Muslim doctors for malpractice, a fact that adds an interesting ethical concern for Muslim patients and those who treat them since the amounts proscribed by Sacred Law are significantly less than some of the common settlements in the West. While consent releases the clinician from responsibility from any unforeseen complications, a physician is nonetheless considered liable for any harmful mistake or procedure performed beyond the scope of his capacity and experience.

Ethical concerns related to clinical practice

Patient confidentiality

One of the most important aspects of professional help is trust between the one seeking the help and the provider, particularly sensitive given the intimate nature of a patient-client relationship. In Islamic Law, all the information necessary for diagnoses and treatment provided by a patient to the physician is considered a sacred trust. The Qur'an speaks of 'Those whose contracts and trusts they vigilantly guard',[8] a description which Dr Qais Al-Mubarak in his legal text on medical issues in Islam says 'includes the trust a physician must honour concerning the treatment of his patients and the secrets they reveal to him'.[9]

Undressing

For Muslims, undressing for physical examinations can be a difficult issue. Islam prescribes a dress code for both men and women, and exposing one's private areas, in particular, is reserved in Islamic Law only for one's spouse. Yet scholars agree that doctors are permitted to see what is necessary. As in the above mentioned categories, the necessity overrules the prescribed dress code.

Patient permission for procedures

According to Muslim jurists, a physician must have permission from a patient or from the guardian of that patient before any medical procedure can be performed. The Maliki jurist Ibn Farhun writes in his authoritative legal text *Tabsirat al-Hukkam*, 'Once a man gives a physician permission to treat him or to circumcise his child, or a veterinarian [permission] to treat his animals, and thereafter loss of life or limb occurs, the physician, if acting prudently, is not liable.'[10] Imam Sarkhusi says, 'because permission is given for a medical procedure, any unforeseeable complications that occur are not indemnified by the physician'.[11]

Patient rights and responsibilities

The right to rescue

In Islamic Law, a human right exists known as *haqq al-is'aaf*, or the right to be rescued, which means that anyone who is able to save a person is obliged to do so, and if he does not, he is held legally liable. This means that a Muslim physician is obliged to treat a person in need of that treatment irrespective of the person's ability to pay the fees.[12]

The right to refuse treatment

The scholars disagree about a patient's right to refuse treatment. The majority of traditional scholars viewed medical treatment as permissible in cases of chronic illness and an obligation in cases of emergency in which loss of life would occur if the person was not treated, such as when haemorrhaging. The traditional scholars, like modern physicians, differentiated between acute, chronic and terminal illnesses. Terminal illness was of particular concern because of inheritance laws as people are not allowed to give more than a third of their wealth away once they have been diagnosed with a terminal illness (the reason behind this law being the prevention of harmful effects that this sometimes has on the ill person's inheritors).

Scholars grouped life threatening illnesses, such as cancer or diabetes, under three classifications. The first type is an illness that has a recognised cure with a high probability of success. According to the majority of jurists, a person has a choice to refuse this treatment. However, the Shafi' school of scholars, one of four authoritative Sunni schools, considered refusing treatment to be a sin, believing that treatment in such a case was a religious obligation, an opinion many modern Muslim scholars have inclined towards. The second type is where there is a probability of success in the treatment, but the treatment's likelihood of success is not particularly high. In this case, scholars generally consider it acceptable to refuse treatment. The third type is an illness considered incurable by most physicians and for which only experimental treatment exists. The majority of scholars discourage treatment in this situation, and some even consider it prohibited. About this third category, Imam al-Ghazzali, an 11th century jurist, says, 'As for illness that leaves little hope of cure, then trusting in providence enjoins leaving any attempt at treating it, and it is this category that the Prophet, peace be upon him, was thinking of when he praised those who left treatment relying on their Lord.'[13]

Each of the four authoritative Sunni schools has differed about the legal ruling of medical treatment. The Hanafi scholars differ among themselves, most regarding treatment to be permissible, including Imam Abu Hanifa himself who Imam An-Nasafi relates to have 'considered medical treatment highly recommended and approximated it to an obligation'.[14] Imam Dardir quotes the authoritative Maliki position regarding the matter, saying, 'Medical treatment, both internal and external, is permissible for anything that medical science deems useful.'[15] The Shafi' school, on the other hand, generally considers it only recommended to seek medical help, which the well-known scholar Imam Nawawi confirms.[16] As mentioned earlier, however, there are those within the school, such as the authoritative Shafi' scholar of the 12th century Imam Baghawi, who see it as an obligation if a cure is likely. In the Hanbali school, medical treatment is permissible, but avoiding it, trusting in God alone for a healing, is considered even better. The Hanbali Imam al-Maruzi states that 'medical treatment is a dispensation but leaving it is a higher spiritual station'.[17] While this is often misunderstood among more devout Muslims as being encouraged, the majority of scholars considered this to be preferable only when the means were not highly efficacious. If treatment has proven to be effective, Muslims are indeed encouraged and in some cases obliged to seek them out.

As for pre-empting illness with preventative medical treatment, most scholars considered it discouraged. However, the authoritative Maliki jurist Abu Bakr ibn al-Arabi said, 'If someone finds an illness or has reason to believe he will be afflicted with it, then it is permissible for him to remove its cause with medical treatment because removing a cause is analogous to removing the thing itself.'[18]

Conclusions

The Prophet Muhammad tells us to 'Seek medical help, for surely God did not send any disease down except that He sent with it a cure.' Throughout history, Muslims have done just this. Moreover, through their legal traditions they have sought to look at the practice of medicine through the light of revealed scriptures and tradition. And through rational reasoning and logical principles, Muslims have created a system whereby present and future ethical questions can be answered. Groups of jurist councils such as the European Fiqh Council in England and the Fiqh Council of North America in the United States are today doing just that. While scholars will continue to differ, the responses emerging from these groups will play an important role in the lives of many devout Muslims seeking medical help today and into the future.

Summary

- Islam champions the pursuit of science and learning and it is thus unsurprising that most Muslims have always been receptive to advances in medicinal progress, be these in the realms of diagnostics, therapeutics or disease monitoring.
- All actions are considered acceptable unless they are explicitly prohibited or contradict any established principles of Islamic Law.
- The Islamic legal methodology is rational and not arbitrary; its principles are therefore relatively easy to understand and apply.

•◦ This does not, however, mean that there are no differences in interpretation. On the contrary, interpretation is a human activity and differences therefore can and do exist. When correctly understood, such differences in views are considered a hallmark of a healthy progressive society.

References

1 Related by Ibn Majah, Ibn Hibban, and Imam al-Hakim.
2 Ibn Khaldun, trans. Franz Rosenthal (1967) *Muqadimma*, p. 387. Bollingen series, Princeton University Press: London.
3 Related by Ibn Majah, Ibn Hibban, and Imam al-Hakim.
4 Al-Jauziya IQ (1999) *Healing with the Medicine of the Prophet*, p. 18. Darussalam: Riyadh, Saudi Arabia.
5 Qur'an, 7:32.
6 As to be expected, there is some difference of opinion on this particular ruling.
7 Al-Qarafi S (1996) *Al-Farooq*, vol. 2, pp. 334–5. Ministry of Endowments: Morocco.
8 Qur'an, 23:8.
9 Al-Mubarak Q (1997) *At-Tadaawi, Masuuliyyah Tibbiyya*, p. 247. Muassat Rayyan: Riyadh, Saudi Arabia.
10 Ibn Farhun, *Tabsirat al-Hukkam*, vol. 2, p. 243. Dar al-Fikr: Beirut.
11 Ibid., p. 231.
12 Bin Bayyah A (2003) *Hiwaar 'an b'ud*, p. 30. Dar al-Andalus al-Khadra: Jeddah.
13 Ghazzali AH (1996) *Ihya 'Ulum ad-Din*, vol. 4, p. 283. Dar al-M'arifah: Beirut.
14 *Majallah Zaytuniyya*, vol. 2, sec. 7, p. 301. Tunis.
15 Ad-Dardir AB (1985) *Sharh as-Saghir*, vol. 4, p. 771. Ministry of Endowments: Abu Dhabi, U.A.E.
16 Nawawi Y (1956) *Al-Minhaj*, vol. 1, p. 344. Matba'at Mustapha Babi al-Halabi: Egypt.
17 Al-Maruzi, quoted in Al-Mubarak Q (1997) *At-Tadaawi, Masuuliyyah Tibbiyya*, vol. 2, p. 357. Muassat Rayyan: Riyadh, Saudi Arabia.
18 Ibn al-Arabi AB, *Al-Qabas*, p. 165. Dar Gharb al-Islami: Beirut.

The Muslim Patient

CHAPTER 5

The family: predicament and promise

(★ *Sangeeta Dhami and Aziz Sheikh*

We live in an era in which the nature, function and structure of the family have been thrown into question. Many, for example, would consider an unmarried couple, a single mother, and same-sex couples as equally legitimate expressions of the family unit. Islam takes a more conservative stance, arguing that the family is a divinely inspired institution, with marriage at its core. In this chapter, we explore what the family means for Muslims living in minority communities in the West. Our aim is not to be prescriptive, but rather to provide clinicians with key insights needed to allow their Muslim patients' concerns to be adequately heard. These concerns, we argue, will often need to be understood in the context of the wider picture, in order to minimise the risk of serious misunderstanding. Case histories are used to illustrate key points.

Family life

One of the most striking features of Muslim society is the importance attached to the family. The family unit is regarded as the cornerstone of a healthy and balanced society.[1] The different plane of emphasis from that found in individual-centred cultures is for many remarkable.

Parental rights

On joining the Muslim community, I was astonished that so much emphasis was put on my relationship with my parents. Here are a few sayings of Muhammad on this subject to which I was exposed almost immediately:

'May his nose be rubbed in the dust! May his nose be rubbed in the dust!' (An Arabic expression denoting degradation). When the Prophet was asked whom he meant by this, he said, 'The one who sees his parents, one or both, during their old age but does not enter Paradise (by doing good to them).'

'A man came to Muhammad and asked his permission to go to battle. The Prophet asked him, "Are your parents alive?" The man replied, "Yes." The Prophet responded, "Then strive to serve them."'[2]

Muslim families: nuclear or extended?

The traditional Muslim family is extended, often spanning three or more generations.[3] An extended structure offers many advantages, including stability, coherence, and physical and psychological support, particularly in times of need.

In Muslim culture, akin to other traditional cultures, respect and esteem increase with age. Elderly parents are respected on account of their life experiences and their hierarchic position within the family unit. The opportunity to attend to the needs of one's parents in their later years is viewed as a gift from Allah.

Support networks

A 28-year-old woman consulted with a physician because of many 'aches' and 'pains', suggesting a strong psychological component to her symptoms. When her notes were reviewed, it transpired that she had had three consecutive stillbirths, the last being only six months previously at 36 weeks' gestation. The possibility of the stillbirths contributing to her current condition was raised. She acknowledged this, saying that she had been coping well while in Pakistan because there she had the support of her extended family. On returning to England, however, she found herself more isolated and was struggling to cope. The option of counselling was discussed but was strongly declined. 'What has happened to me is a test from Allah and something I will come to terms with. Counsellors cannot understand this.'

Challenges to the extended family

In practice, it is usual for a new bride to move into the household of her husband. The change is often considerable, and problems in the fledgling relationship between the bride and her in-laws are common. This transition is all the more difficult where Muslims live as minorities because, in many cases, migration patterns have resulted in fragmentation of the extended family structure. Many second- and third-generation Muslim migrants have grown up in nuclear families, not having first-hand familiarity with the richness and complexity of living within extended family networks. In addition, despite religious teachings that encourage marriage at an early age, a secular trend to marry late is being seen among Muslims.

Some observers have suggested that increasing age curtails a person's ability to adapt to change, adaptability being the hallmark of youth. Finally, and perhaps most important of all, Muslim youth in the West are faced with lifestyle choices not available in more traditional cultures. To some, the opportunities with respect to individual freedom offered by a nuclear family structure far outweigh any benefits of living in an extended family.[3]

Discharging responsibilities

An elderly Bengali man was recovering in a hospital from an episode of pneumonia. He was bed-bound, the result of multiple strokes. On the geriatric team's prompting, the family was approached by social services to discuss a nursing home placement. The family explained that they would prefer to look after him at home. With the support of his physician and social services, he was able to stay in the family home until his death a few years later.

The challenge of ageing

'Things are not like they used to be. There is an increasing trickle of Muslims entering nursing homes, and I've actually been thinking of opening a home specifically for Muslims.'

– Muslim nursing home proprietor

Gender and segregation

Gender issues and, in particular, the rights of women in Muslim culture, continue to generate much media attention in the West. Muslim women are often portrayed as inferior beings, desperately in need of liberation from the Muslim patriarchal culture that prevents their progress. Segregation of the sexes, a practice encouraged by Islam, is often seen as proof of the suppression of Muslim women.[4] Although certainly much can be done to improve the position of women in Muslim culture, the stereotype created in the Western media leaves much to be desired. Such misunderstandings are largely due to naive and simplistic attempts to transpose a Western set of norms and values onto women with a very different history and culture. A detailed critique of the feminist position is beyond the scope of this article; readers are referred to other texts.[5,6]

Any questions?

At a seminar on transcultural medicine, junior physicians were asked if they had any particular questions about Islam. Anonymous responses were encouraged to allow the physicians to raise issues of genuine concern without fear of offending the group leader (a Muslim). Two themes dominated: women's rights and fundamentalism.

As already noted, Islam clearly demarcates between legitimate and illegitimate human relationships. Societal laws exist to aid Muslims in abiding by this framework. Segregation, therefore, exists primarily to minimise the chances of illicit relationships developing. Physical contact between members of the opposite sex is strongly discouraged, although these rules are relaxed somewhat if medical treatment is required.[7] This framework explains why many prefer to see a same-sex clinician, particularly in consultations necessitating examination of the genitalia. On a practical note, if recourse to an interpreter is required, the use of same-sex interpreters offers a considerable advantage. The issue of gender segregation is one that should also be considered when planning health education campaigns, research interviews and similar ventures.

Barbed wire

Zara, a 27-year-old housewife from Sudan, attended for a follow-up appointment at her local hospital. Her physician was on leave, so she was seen by a locum replacement. On entering the patient's room, the physician extended his hand. Zara politely declined, but failed to give her reasons for doing so. The resulting consultation was tense and dysfunctional.

Gender and role demarcation

The man is considered the head of the family; to many a man, however, this is a poisoned chalice because with leadership comes responsibility. Economic responsibility for maintaining the family falls squarely on the shoulders of the man, irrespective of whether his wife is earning. Unemployment, then, can greatly affect the integrity of the family, leaving the man in a role limbo. Psychological morbidity in such situations may be high, with ramifications for the family as a whole.

Marriage

> You are a garment to them, and they are a garment for you.
>
> – *Qur'an*[8]

You earn too much!

Mrs Mu'min attended as an 'extra' towards the end of a busy morning surgery. An accountant, she was the principal breadwinner and brought home a healthy wage. Her husband, a doctor trained in Somalia, was unable to practise his craft because his qualifications were not recognised in the United Kingdom. During the last three years, he had been forced into various manual occupations. The reason for her consultation? Confused, distraught, and visibly shaken, she explained that her husband was threatening to leave her unless she gave up her job.

This succinct Qur'anic simile encapsulates the primary aims of marriage – to provide warmth, comfort and protection, and to beautify. Within the Islamic vision, children have a right to be conceived and reared in a stable and secure environment; marriage is deemed to provide such an environment. In contrast, celibacy and sex outside of marriage are strongly discouraged because they are considered behavioural extremes that are not conducive to a wholesome society.[9]

In many senses, marriage is considered the union of two families, and the parents usually arrange the marriage. Although the free consent of both the bride and groom are essential, parental coercion is often strong.

Some parents are evidently beginning to understand the marital concerns of their children. The practice of choosing marriage partners from within one's community, however, continues to be considered important by young and old.

Consanguinity

Consanguinity (intermarriage) is particularly common in Muslims of South Asian, Turkish and Arab origin. Among British Pakistani Muslims, current estimates are that some 75% of couples are in a consanguineous relationship, and approximately 50% are married to first cousins. This represents an increase from the generation of their parents, of whom only 30% are married to first cousins.[10,11] Consanguinity confers many advantages, which, at least in part, explain its continued appeal. For example, it allows a thorough knowledge of the future marriage partner for sons or daughters – a particularly important consideration in Muslim minority communities where the usual social networks that facilitate the search for an appropriate partner may be lacking.

Whereas consanguinity doubtless results in an increased frequency of familial disorders with an autosomal recessive pattern of inheritance,[12] assessing the relative contribution of consanguinity to the high rates of congenital defect and perinatal mortality among Pakistanis is far from easy. Other factors of importance in the birth outcome debate include the high prevalence of deprivation among Muslims, difficulties with access to high-quality genetic and prenatal counselling, and the possible risks associated with culturally insensitive maternity care.[13,14] Appropriate services specifically tailored to meet the needs of Muslims and other minority groups should be considered an issue deserving priority attention.

Sex, menstruation and contraception

Sexual norms

Sex in the context of marriage is a legitimate, enjoyable activity – an act of worship that is deserving of Allah's reward. Conversely, sex outside of heterosexual marriage is considered deviant, deserving of punishment in the hereafter. In keeping with orthodox Judeo-Christian teaching, homosexuality is considered sinful. A distinction is made, however, between a homosexual inclination and the act itself. The former is acceptable so long as it is not practised.[15]

Promiscuity does exist among Muslims, although in all probability its prevalence is considerably lower than in some segments of Western society.[16] Those who operate outside the Muslim framework often find themselves ostracised and held responsible for bringing the family name into disrepute. The prospect of 'coming out' for homosexual Muslims is, therefore, not realistic at present.

Despite the positive outlook towards sex, it is not a subject that is openly discussed. Cultural taboos dictate that sex should remain a private matter between husband and wife. This explains, at least in part, why Muslims are often reluctant to seek help for sexual problems and the long time lag before seeing a physician.

Menstruation

While menstruating, women are exempt from some of the important religious rites, such as ritual prayer, fasting and *Hajj* (the pilgrimage to Mecca). Sexual intercourse is also prohibited at such times. All other forms of physical contact between husband and wife, such as hugging and kissing, are allowed. Menstruation, therefore, may have many social and psychological ramifications. There are also many possible implications for clinical care. Women may be reluctant to see a physician for gynaecological symptoms, cervical smear tests, or intrauterine device checks for fear of bleeding following a pelvic examination. Many Muslim women are unaware that traumatic bleeding of this kind is distinct from menstrual bleeding and, hence, the religious constraints do not apply. Education is needed both within the Muslim community and among professionals so that the importance and implications of genital tract bleeding are better appreciated.

Women may consult their physician or family planning clinic to postpone their menstrual periods at particular times. The most common situation is in the period before *Hajj*. For those using the combined oral contraceptive pill, they can be safely advised to either 'bicycle' or 'tricycle' pill packs. This involves omitting the seven-day break between pill packs, thus avoiding the withdrawal bleeding that ensues.[17] Alternatively, progesterone (for example, norethisterone [norethindrone]) may be used daily, beginning two to three days before the period is due and continuing treatment until such time that bleeding is more convenient.

Additional dimensions in the management of genital tract bleeding

A married woman in her late thirties contacted a friend (a female Muslim physician) to discuss her menstrual problems. She had been bleeding on a fortnightly basis for the previous few months. This was causing havoc with prayer routines because on each occasion she had stopped praying. She was advised that she should continue praying because the pattern of bleeding was unlikely to represent menstrual bleeding. It was suggested that she see her physician for further investigation. Thus far, she had avoided consultation. Contributing to her apprehension were the prospect of not being able to see a woman physician, difficulties in articulating the real reason for her attendance, and the possibility that an internal examination may exacerbate her bleeding.

Female genital tract mutilation

Female genital tract mutilation is a practice that is carried out in many regions of the world, including some Muslim countries. This practice is most widespread in parts of Africa, stretching in a band from the Horn through Central Africa and extending to parts of Nigeria.[18] The custom's exact origins are uncertain, but it almost certainly predates the arrival of Christianity and Islam to these regions. Female genital mutilation is currently illegal in many countries, including Britain.[19]

The procedure has different forms and is typically done at the age of six or seven years. The least invasive of these involves removing only the prepuce of the clitoris. Removal of the clitoris, or more extensive procedures, is not approved by religious teaching; nonetheless, these extreme practices continue in some Muslim regions largely because of the strong influences of tribal and regional custom and tradition. The most extreme form, infibulation, involves excising the clitoris, the labia minora, and the medial aspect of the labia majora. The sides of the vagina are then sutured, leaving a small opening for the passage of urine and menstrual flow.[20] An intermediate form involves removing the clitoris either partially or totally, together with a portion of the labia minora.

The removal of large amounts of genital tissue can cause considerable problems, including difficulties with micturation, recurrent urinary tract infection, dyspareunia, and dysmenorrhoea. The emotional and psychological ramifications of such bodily assaults are also now being appreciated.

Traditionally, a local midwife performs a deinfibulation immediately after marriage, thus allowing consummation to occur. The recent large-scale migration from Somalia, Sudan, Eritrea and Ethiopia to parts of Europe has highlighted the difficulties and problems involved with caring for infibulated women. Access to deinfibulation is restricted in the United Kingdom, and women will, therefore, often become pregnant while infibulated, hindering their care in pregnancy and in labour.

Contraception

Many traditions of the Prophet Muhammad extol the merits of marriage, procreation and fecundity.[21] Muslim opinion with respect to contraception is divided, a minority arguing that it is categorically prohibited whereas the majority opinion is that contraception is allowed but discouraged.[22] A small minority, confined largely to academic circles, suggests that effective family planning strategies are essential to prevent the global overspill predicted by many in the West.[23] The prevalence of contraceptive use in Muslim countries varies widely, reflecting these divergent views, and ranges from less than 5% (in Mauritania, North Yemen, Somalia and Sudan) to more than 50% (in Turkey, Lebanon and Tunisia).[24]

Summary

- The family forms the basic building block of Muslim society. Despite the many pressures it faces, the family institution remains strong. The future of the extended family, however, is under considerable threat.
- Marriage forms the sole basis for sexual relations and parenthood.
- Islamic Law generally discourages the use of contraception, extolling the virtues of large families, but there seems to be a trend toward smaller families.
- Some social problems such as sexually transmitted infections, cervical cancer and unwanted pregnancies may be mitigated by developing vehicles to strengthen the traditional Muslim family structure.
- Female genital mutilation is common among Muslim and non-Muslim women of African origin.

References

1 Doi AR (1984) *Shar'iah: the Islamic Law*, pp. 114–27. Ta Ha: London.
2 Lang J (1995) *Struggling to Surrender*, p. 133. Amana: Maryland.
3 Anwar M (1994) *Young Muslims in Britain: attitudes, educational needs, and policy implications*. Islamic Foundation: Leicester.
4 Goodwin J (1995) *Price of Honour*. Warner: London.
5 Waddy C (1980) *Women in Muslim History*. Longman: London.
6 Badawi JA (1997) *Woman: under the shade of Islam*. El-Falah: Cairo.
7 McDermott MY, Ahsan MM (1993) *The Muslim Guide*. Islamic Foundation: Leicester.
8 Ali YA (1938) *The Meaning of the Glorious Quran*; **2**: 187. Dar al-Kitab: Cairo (translation modified).
9 Al-Qaradawi Y (1990) *The Lawful and the Prohibited in Islam*, pp.148–236. American Trust Publications: Indianapolis.
10 Darr A, Modell B (1988) The frequency of consanguineous marriage among British Pakistanis. *J Med Genet*; **25**: 186–90.
11 Gatrad AR, Sheikh A (2005) Success in tackling deafness with multi-faceted interventions. *Arch Dis Child*; **90**: 443–4.

12 Bundey S, Alam H, Kaur A, Mir S, Lancashire RJ (1990) Race, consanguinity and social features in Birmingham babies: a basis for prospective study. *J Epidemiol Community Health*; **44**: 130–5.

13 Bowler I (1993) 'They're not the same as us?': midwives' stereotype of south Asian maternity patients. *Social Health Illness*; **15**: 157–78.

14 Sivagnanman R (2004) *Experience of Maternity Services: Muslim women's perspectives*. The Maternity Alliance: London.

15 Wayte C (1999). Bible is disapproving of homosexual activity but not homosexual orientation [letter]. *BMJ*; **319**: 123–4.

16 Francome C (1994) *The Great Leap 2: a study of Muslim students*. Middlesex University: London.

17 Guillebaud J (1991) *The Pill*. Oxford University Press: Oxford.

18 Dorkenoo E (1994) *Cutting the Rose*. Minority Rights Publication: London.

19 Black JA, Debelle GD (1995) Female genital mutilation in Britain. *BMJ*; **310**: 1590–2.

20 Keller NHM (1997) *Reliance of the Traveller*. Amana: Maryland.

21 Hasan S (1998) *Raising Children in Islam*. Al Quran Society: London.

22 Ebrahim AFM (1998) *Abortion, Birth Control and Surrogate Parenting: an Islamic perspective*. American Trust Publications: Indianapolis.

23 Rahman F (1998) *Health and Medicine in the Islamic Tradition*. Kazi: Chicago.

24 Oberneger CM (1994) Reproductive choices in Islam: gender and state in Iran and Tunisia. *Stud Fam Plann*; **25**: 41–51.

CHAPTER 6

Birth customs: meaning and significance

(★ *Abdul Rashid Gatrad and Aziz Sheikh*

Muslims are now being born in the West in significant numbers.[1] The overwhelming majority of Muslims in Europe and North America, and indeed globally, will respect the rites of passage recommended by Islamic teaching. Despite the sizes of these Muslim communities, and the importance attached to birth customs by them, few healthcare professionals will have received any formal training in transcultural perspectives and customs surrounding birth. This chapter intends to begin the process of bridging this gap with respect to Muslims. The customs are many, and to the uninitiated may seem unnecessarily rigid and prescriptive – to those within the tradition they are, however, deeply symbolic, coherent and complementary. Above all, they serve to remind the new parents that a fresh chapter is about to unfold in their personal and collective narratives. To fully appreciate the joy, richness, honour and potential of parenthood there is a constant need to look beyond the material dimensions of life.

The rights of the child

> O My Lord! Grant unto me from Thee a progeny that is pure:
> for thou art He that heareth prayer.
>
> *– Qur'an*[2]

The child's rights over his parents are clearly articulated in Sacred Law. For the most part these are well respected by Muslim parents. These rights begin before conception, stemming back to the all-important choice of marriage partner.

Does a child have rights over his father?

A man once came to Umar (the second Caliph of Islam) complaining of his son's disobedience. Umar called for the boy, and asked him about his father's complaint, and his neglect of his duties towards his father. The boy replied:

'O Caliph! Does a child not have rights over his father?'

'Certainly,' replied Umar.

'What are they then?' enquired the boy.

'That he should choose his mother with care, preferring a righteous woman. When Allah blesses him with a child, he should give him a good name and teach him the Qur'an.'

'O Caliph! My father did none of these. My mother was a fire-worshipper. He gave me the name Ju'laan (meaning dung beetle) and did not teach me a single letter of the Qur'an.'

Turning to the father Umar said, 'You have come to me to complain about the disobedience of your son. You have failed in your duty to him before he has failed in his duty to you; you have done wrong to him before he has wronged you.'[3]

Children have the right to be born through a legitimate union, with full knowledge of their parentage. The social experiments currently taking place in some countries facilitating the use of donor sperms and eggs to help barren couples to conceive is, for this and other reasons, categorically prohibited by Islam. They also have the right to a good name, to be suckled, educated and, above all, to have a loving and caring environment in which they may thrive to fulfil their Allah-given potential. 'Paradise lies at the feet of your mother' is a Prophetic maxim, emphasising the unique standing of our first relationship, that will be recognised by Muslims the world over.

Whither the extended family

'It is a matter of sadness that many children are denied the benefits of not having a grandparent to cherish and dote on them, to take them back on journeys back in time and spin yarns for them. We say again that the trend towards nuclear families is a trend for the impoverishment of children.'

– Abdul Wahid Hamid[4]

Birth customs

The Adhan

It is only proper that the first word that a baby should hear is the name of his creator, Allah. This is to be followed by the Declaration of Faith, '*There is no deity but Allah; Muhammad is the Messenger of Allah.*' Both of these fundamental pronouncements serve as the pivot around which the life of a Muslim rotates, hence their symbolic significance at birth. Both pronouncements are conveniently encapsulated within the call to prayer, or *Adhan*.

The father whispers the *Adhan* into the baby's right ear, serving as a reminder that the father also has a key responsibility in the months and years ahead. Ideally, this should be as soon as possible after birth. The entire ceremony takes only a few minutes, and it is greatly appreciated if parents are allowed the opportunity to perform this rite in privacy.

The *Adhan* ceremony in many ways serves as a metaphor for life itself. Those that have had the opportunity of witnessing a Muslim congregational prayer will be aware that shortly after the *Adhan*, and immediately preceding the prayer, there is a second shorter call to prayer. This second call is the *Iqamah* (Figure 6.1). At the time of birth there is an *Adhan* but no *Iqamah*. For the funeral prayer, however, there is simply the *Iqamah* with no preceding *Adhan*. Our stay on earth is short – the equivalent of the few minutes separating the *Adhan* from the *Iqamah* – so life then should be spent wisely and diligently, and not wasted.

FIGURE 6.1 Diagrammatic representation of the relationship between the Adhan, Iqamah and Prayer

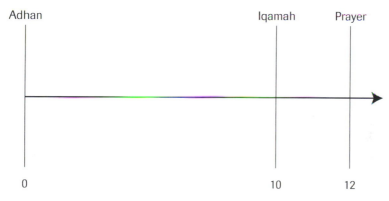

Time (minutes)

Tahneek

This is a commonly observed practice, which, like many of the others mentioned in this chapter, traces its origins back to the Prophet Muhammad. Soon after birth, and preferably before being fed, a small piece of softened date is gently rubbed into the infant's upper palate. Where dates are not easily available, substitutes such as honey are used. A respected member of the family often performs this, with the hope that some of his positive qualities will be transmitted to the fledgling infant. The practice of only permitting access to partners into the delivery ward has its advantages, but may be seen by some as unduly restrictive, impeding the practice of this custom.[5]

Taweez

A *Taweez* is a piece of black string, with a small pouch containing a prayer, which is tied around the baby's wrist or neck. It is particularly common among Muslims from the Indian subcontinent, with many believing that it protects the baby from ill health. For obvious reasons, it is important that the *Taweez* be handled with respect, and should not be removed or broken except during emergency treatment.

Circumcision

Despite the fact that an estimated one-third of the global male population is circumcised, the issue of male religious circumcision continues to excite a good deal of interest and discussion both within the medical and lay press. Sharply conflicting customs are seen in Western countries, with circumcision being performed on an almost routine basis in the USA,[6] whereas in many parts of Europe it is a practice viewed by many with suspicion and scorn.[7,8] Although not often enquired about, the Muslim view appears pretty clear that this should ideally be a state run service.[9] Elsewhere we have discussed at length the ethics and legality of religious circumcision considering this question in the light of the recent European Human Rights Act and also considered models for state provision, including those in which the user of such services pays, thus rendering the scheme safer than the current often poorly unregulated provision and also cost-neutral to the state.[10,11]

For Muslims,[11] as for their Jewish brethren,[12] religious law sanctions male circumcision. Female circumcision is discussed in an earlier chapter (Chapter 5). Circumcision is considered particularly important for hygiene purposes, as when the child matures and begins to offer prayers, there is no danger of his clothes becoming soiled from small amounts of urine 'held up' in the foreskin – important because soiled clothes will nullify the prayer. Despite the recent attempts of some Muslim apologists to downplay the importance of circumcision,[13] it seems highly probable that it will continue, particularly in view of the publication of recent high quality experimental studies confirming its health benefits.[14,15]

Difficulties involved with obtaining state circumcision in Britain necessitate that it is usually performed in the private sector, at a cost of between £50 and £100. The plastic ring method is most often used, with the procedure performed under a local anaesthetic. Though most practitioners seem to be aware of the need to delay circumcision in jaundiced infants, because of the risk of prolonged bleeding, it is important to remind parents of this. Babies born with hypospadias should also avoid circumcision until a surgical opinion has been sought.[16] Because of the frequency of complications following circumcision by non-professionals, some health authorities have tried to regulate the practice by establishing special clinics for religious circumcision.[17] Others, such as Sandwell Health Authority in the UK, have gone one step further, offering free circumcision to males under the age of two years.[18] Such initiatives are very welcome, and deserve to be replicated in other areas as the question of pain is addressed and bleeding minimised.[10]

In the nick of time!

A two-week-old baby was brought into the accident & emergency department by his anxious parents, concerned that he was becoming increasingly listless. Further questioning revealed that he had been circumcised some 24 hours earlier. Since then he had been bleeding steadily from his circumcision wound. On examination he was peripherally shut down, with a haemoglobin count of only 5.5 g/dl.

He was resuscitated, the haemorrhage arrested and an emergency blood transfusion arranged. A private practitioner had performed the circumcision. No follow-up had been arranged, and the parents had been given no advice about possible complications.

There were no National Health Service facilities for religious circumcision in the area.

Although usually performed on the seventh day, it is common in some communities to delay the procedure for a few months or years. Bengali communities often delay the circumcision for a few months in summer born babies, preferring the winter period, as wound healing is believed to be better. Frequent nappy changes should be advised, together with the liberal use of barrier creams, in order to minimise the risk of ammoniacal dermatitis and the associated risks of meatal stenosis and ulceration while wound healing occurs.[19,20] Turkish Muslim communities may wait until just before puberty.

Aqiqah

A sheep is offered in sacrifice for every newborn child as a sign of one's gratitude to Allah. This is usually also performed on the seventh day and the meat distributed among family members and the poor. Many will arrange for the sacrifice to be performed in their countries of origin, thus allowing the meat to be distributed where there is greater need, while simultaneously enabling disparate family members to partake in the celebrations.

Shaving the hair

A newborn child is innocent, free from the internal failings that grip the majority of humankind – the diseases of avarice, lust, envy and pride, to mention but a few. As a symbolic act, the scalp hair that grew during intrauterine development are removed, traditionally on the seventh day of life, and the equivalent weight in silver is given in charity. There is another point in time that the Muslim has the opportunity to re-enter this noble state of innocence. The Prophet likened the one that successfully emerges from the standing on the desert plane of Arafat during Hajj (Chapter 8), having beseeched Allah's forgiveness for past excesses, as pure, 'like the day his mother gave him birth'. The pilgrim is asked to remove his scalp hair to commemorate this accomplishment.

Muslim names

Choosing a name

As has already been noted, the choice of a good name is one of the basic rights of a child. It is hoped that the name will both inspire self-respect and give the child something to aspire towards in the years that lie ahead. After birth it may be a few days before the child is named, as it is usual to seek the advice, and approval, of members of the extended family. Some examples of common female and male names, together with their meanings, are presented in Tables 6.1 and 6.2.

TABLE 6.1 Examples of common female names and their meanings

FEMALE NAMES	MEANING
Aminah	Trustworthy, faithful
Faridah	Unique
Fatimah	The Prophet's daughter
Nafisa	Precious
Rabiah	Garden
Salma	Peaceful

TABLE 6.2 Examples of common male names and their meanings

MALE NAMES	MEANING
Abdullah	Servant of Allah
Ahmed	Praiseworthy
Hamza	The Prophet's uncle
Musa	Moses
Sa'eed	Happy
Tahir	Pure

What's his name?

A young couple was keen to name their first-born Abdul-Khaliq (meaning 'Servant of the Creator'). All family members agreed that the name was pleasant and gave much to aspire towards. There was, however, at the same time a degree of apprehension on the part of some that the name would be 'ruined' by those who failed to appreciate its significance, being either mispronounced or shortened to Abdul (meaning 'Servant'). After a few days of trying the name the family's anxieties were confirmed. The name Yusuf (Joseph) was chosen as an alternative – a choice that was met with widespread approval.

Naming systems

It is in Gujarati Muslim communities, and among Muslims who have their origins in Central Africa and in urban regions of the Indian subcontinent, that the system of naming often follows that found in the West. Families will use clan or group names as a surname, such as Khan or Chaudhry. For many Muslims, however, a more traditional method of naming is used, and it is usually a failure to understand this system that leads to confusion, and occasionally chaos, with medical records.

Boys may have a personal name, which is either preceded or followed by a religious title, such as Muhammad Siddiq, where Muhammad is a religious title and Siddiq the personal name. In the case of his brother, Altaf Hussain, Altaf is the personal name and Hussain (the name of a grandson of the Prophet) the title. For medical records, the final name is often used as a surname and this would explain why two Muslim brothers might have different surnames! A possible alternative method of recording family names is to use the child's personal name followed by his father's personal name – the latter being used as a surname, such as Muhammad Siddiq and Altaf Hussain, the sons of Abdul Rashid, would be recorded as Siddiq Rashid and Altaf Rashid, since Abdul is a title. There are only a handful of titles commonly used; therefore such a system could be implemented with relatively little training required for record clerks. The potential problems posed by using different names on hospital records and other important documentation, such as passports, driving licences and insurance forms, to mention but a few, would, however, need to be thoroughly explored in advance of any such changes. Anecdotal discussions suggest that there would not be much resistance among Muslims to a change of this kind; nonetheless, it is clearly important that the views of a representative group from the Muslim community are adequately sought.

Many Pakistani and Bangladeshi Muslim women will use a personal name, followed by a title, such as Razia Bibi or Razia Begum, where Razia is the personal name and Bibi and Begum are titles denoting marital status (Miss or Mrs). A similar practice could be adopted for recording female names; that is, their personal name followed by their father's or husband's personal name. Razia Begum, the wife of Abdul Rashid, could then be recorded as Razia Rashid (Table 6.3).

TABLE 6.3 Traditional Muslim naming system and a proposed alternative recording system for use in UK medical records

FAMILY MEMBER	NAME	RECORDED AS
Husband	Abdul Rashid Rahman	Rashid Rahman
Wife	Razia Begum	Razia Rashid
Eldest son	Muhammad Siddiq	Siddiq Rashid
Younger son	Altaf Hussain	Altaf Rashid
Daughter	Mariam Bibi	Mariam Rashid

Some help in recognising Muslim names

Muslims are very adept at recognising the names of other Muslims, easily distinguishing them from those of other faiths. Usually Arabic in origin – the language of the Qur'an – Muslim names are easily identifiable to the trained eye. For those less familiar with Arabic, title names can be very useful in identifying Muslims. Commonly used titles are Muhammad, Hussain, Abdul, Ali, Ahmad, Bibi, Begum and Khatoon, and therefore any individual with a name incorporating one of these titles can confidently be identified as a Muslim.

Sikhism and Hinduism are the two other major religious groupings found among the peoples of the Indian subcontinent. Both groups often have characteristic names that allow religious affiliation to be easily recognised. Common Sikh names include Kaur, Singh, Gill, Samra, Baines, Uppal, Mann, Khera and names ending in -jit or -jeet. Common Hindu names include Ben, Devi, Kumar, Das, Lal and Patel, although Gujrati Muslims also occasionally use Patel.

Breast-feeding and weaning

Breast-feeding

Breast-feeding is positively encouraged by religious teachings; ideally this should continue for a period of two years.[21] Although Muslim mothers may want to breast-feed, the insufficient privacy offered by some postnatal wards is an important barrier. Muslim etiquette requires that women should not expose certain bodily parts to anyone except their husbands. This includes the breasts, and in order to observe this privacy while in hospital, it is often most convenient to bottle-feed. The trouble with this, however, is that milk production may be adversely affected, particularly in cases where prolonged hospital admission has become necessary. There is a commonly held belief among some first-generation migrants that colostrum is either harmful to the baby or that it has poor nutritional value.[22,23] Supplements of honey and water will often be used for the first few days of life.[24] There is no religious basis for this belief. This is an example of a practice that contradicts religious teaching; this dissonance offers a very useful window for the development of educational campaigns directed towards Muslim mothers, with the support of religious leaders and Muslim organisations.

Breast milk from a Muslim mother can be given to another baby but (when older) that baby and his or her mother should be told of this. In religious law, children who receive breast milk from the same person are classed as siblings and therefore, when of age, are prohibited from marrying each other.

Prolonged breast-feeding (longer than six months) is the norm among Bangladeshis.[25] This can lead to iron-deficiency anaemia and rickets if breast-feeding is not supplemented with an appropriately balanced diet. Most south Asian families change from an infant formula to 'doorstep' cow's milk at about five to six months.[24] This is contrary to the UK Department of Health recommendation which states that reconstituted infant formulas should be continued beyond six months in order to prevent deficiencies of iron and vitamins A, C and D.[26]

Weaning

With the exception of Bangladeshis, most Muslim babies are weaned between the age of three and five months. Proprietary tinned foods are most commonly used, probably more a reflection of the poor socio-economic status of many Muslim households, rather than anything to do with religious teaching.[27] Islamic teaching encourages 'wholesome food'[28] and initiatives could, and perhaps should, be developed, using an appropriate cultural framework to encourage greater use of fresh fruits and vegetables during weaning. This is particularly important in view of the high prevalence of caries, diabetes and ischaemic heart disease among Muslims. Importantly, it is worth remembering that babies are often fed by hand, and children may be positively encouraged to hand-feed. Such a child's spoon-handling skills may be poorly developed – something that needs to be borne in mind if using a spoon is incorporated into developmental assessment tests.

The handicapped child

Many children born with handicaps do not survive in developing countries – thus the care of a handicapped child, especially in cases where the disability is severe, is a relatively new experience for Muslim communities. There is, for example, no word in the Urdu language which adequately explains mental or physical retardation. Parents tend to accept the deformity as an act of Allah, some rationalising it as a 'test from Allah' or as a form of retribution for sins that they may have previously committed. This latter perspective may be seen as a blessing, since it is better to be punished in this world than in the eternal abode of the hereafter. A mother may try to make amends and seek help from a religious leader to effect a cure for the handicap or to prevent recurrences. Unfortunately, charlatans are common and the opportunities for exploitation considerable.

Language problems are often a major barrier in the care of handicapped

Muslim children because there is a shortage of multilingual therapists in areas such as occupational therapy, speech therapy and social work. Parental reluctance to participate in group work/therapy may stem from fear that involvement may publicise the child's handicap within the wider community, adversely affecting the marriage prospects of siblings. Self-help Muslim groups are slowly beginning to emerge, and dialogue between such agencies and professional groups is to be encouraged, so as to allow healthcare professionals the opportunity to hear and understand the concerns of minority populations and fine-tune services appropriately.

Deprivation, consanguinity and the general reluctance of Muslims to abort foetuses with congenital anomalies are key reasons for the high levels of handicap found among the Muslim community. Tackling health inequalities remains an important priority for governments, and it is expected that this will in due course bring major health benefits to the deprived. Consanguinity, as discussed in Chapter 5, remains high among certain ethnic groups; for families with a history of congenital anomalies, access to high-quality genetic counselling is essential.[29,30] Where congenital abnormalities are detected during pregnancy, it is important to discuss the possible implications of the findings with the parents (and religious leader if appropriate). This is particularly true for anomalies detected early on in pregnancy, since some jurists hold that termination is acceptable in such circumstances before 'ensoulment' of the foetus occurs – an event that takes place on the 120th day of life.

Using religious beliefs and cultural practices in a 'recipe book' manner can sometimes be used as a shield to avoid difficult and painful discussions. The assumption that since Islamic belief discourages abortion, Muslim parents should not be given the choice of abortion is unfair. Rather, this information should be used as a backdrop against which to explore the wishes of the *individual couple* concerned. Whatever is eventually decided, parents have the right to be supported in their final decision, even if this goes against professional or religious opinion.

Adoption and fostering

Adoption involves conferring to the adopted person the status and rights of a natural son or daughter. From the discussion above, natural offspring have rights that predate conception; they also have rights that extend beyond the lifespan of the parents, for example the right to inherit. According to religious teaching, it is not possible for someone to assume parentage on the basis of a simple declaration; adoption then is considered an attempt to deny reality.[31]

Professional imperialism

A recently married genetics student attended the antenatal 'booking-in' clinic in her first pregnancy. A routine dating ultrasound scan was performed which revealed that the foetus had increased nuchal thickness. Suspecting a diagnosis of Down's syndrome her consultant referred her to a tertiary centre for further investigations. Here she was followed up with serial ultrasound scans. It soon emerged that there were a number of congenital malformations, which were considered to be incompatible with life. She was repeatedly advised to have a termination on the basis that it was thought the baby had a less then 1% chance of survival. This she consistently declined, stating that abortion was against her faith.

Ultrasound monitoring continued until 34 weeks when she spontaneously went into labour. The baby was stillborn. She was named, buried and is visited frequently by family members.

In comparison, foster care, being devoid of the legal implications noted above, is strongly encouraged. Fostering is not uncommon, usually between family members, where following an unplanned pregnancy in an already large family, the infant may be offered to a childless couple. Many first-generation Muslims will themselves have first-hand familiarity with being fostered, often with close relatives following the death of parents. If a Muslim child is to be fostered this needs to be with a Muslim family. The Muslim community usually opposes any suggestions of a Muslim child being placed with those of another faith background very strongly. We suspect that many other religious groups would on the whole express very similar sentiments.

Summary

- The Muslim child has a number of Allah-given rights; these include the right to be born through a legitimate union, to know fully one's parentage, to be suckled, and to be reared with kindness and respect.
- The traditional Muslim naming system often causes confusion with medical records. This naming system can be adapted to allow family members to be readily identified, though the legal implications and possible logistic problems posed by such a change have not yet been assessed.
- There are a number of birth customs common to Muslims. Most healthcare professionals will have received little training in understanding their meaning or significance. An appreciation of such customs provides a unique insight into the lives of many Muslims.
- Male circumcision is an important birth custom. Parents should be advised to delay the procedure in the case of neonatal jaundice and hypospadias. Religious circumcision should be available from state health services.
- Caring for handicapped children is a relatively new experience for many Muslims. Culturally appropriate support services are currently poorly developed.

References

1 Pharoah POD, Alberman ED (1990) Annual statistical review. *Arch Dis Child*; **65**: 147–51.

2 Ali YA (1938) *The Meaning of the Glorious Quran*; **3**: 38 (trans modified). Dar al-Kitab: Cairo.

3 Hasan S (1998) *Raising Children in Islam*, pp. 23–33. Al Quran Society: London.

4 Hamid AW (1989) *Islam the Natural Way*, p. 75. MELS: London.

5 Gatrad AR, Sheikh A (2001) Muslim birth customs. *Arch Dis Child Fetal Neonatal Ed*; **84**: F6–8.

6 Anon (1999) Circumcision policy statement, American Academy of Paediatrics, Task Force on Circumcision. *Paediatrics*; **103**: 686–93.

7 Gairdner D (1949) The fate of the foreskin. *BMJ*; **ii**: 1433–7.

8 Black JA, Debelle GD (1996) Female genital mutilation. *BMJ*; **312**: 377–8.

9 Bhopal R, Madhok R, Hameed A (1998) Religious circumcision on the NHS: opinions of Pakistani people in Middlesbrough, England. *J Epidemiol Commun Hlth*; **52**: 758–9.

10 Gatrad AR, Sheikh A, Jacks H (2002) Religious circumcision and the Human Rights Act. *Arch Dis Child*; **86**: 76–8.

11 Gatrad AR, Khan A, Shafi S, Sheikh A (2005) Promoting safer circumcision for British Muslims. *Diversity in Heath and Social Care*, **2**: 37–40.

12 Spitzer J (1998) *A Guide to the Orthodox Jewish Way of Life for Healthcare Professionals*, pp. 72–3. J Spitzer: London.

13 Siddiqui AR, Dhami S, Ben Hamida F (1999) Complications of circumcision (correspondence). *General Practitioner*; **Nov 13**: 50.

14 Gray RJ, Kigozi G, Serwadda D, *et al.* (2007) Male circumcision for HIV prevention in men in Rakai, Uganda: a randomised trial. *Lancet*; **369**: 657–66.

15 Bailey RC, Moses S, Parker CB, *et al.* (2007). Male circumcision for HIV prevention in young men in Kisumu, Kenya: a randomised controlled trial. *Lancet*; **369**: 643–56.

16 Meadow SR, Smithells RW (1991) *Lecture Notes on Paediatrics*, p. 194. Blackwell: Oxford.

17 Memon M, Prowse M (1999) Joint working. One for the boys. *Hlth Serv J*; **109**: 26–7.

18 Anon (1997) *The Muslim News*, p 85 www.muslimnews.co.uk/santwell.html

19 Dunn DC, Rawlinson N (1991) *Surgical Diagnosis and Management*, p. 448. Blackwell: Oxford.

20 Stenram A, Malmfors G, Okmian L (1986) Circumcision for phymosis: indications and results. *Acta Paediatr Scand*; **75**: 321–3.

21 Ali YA (1938) *The Meaning of the Glorious Quran*; **2**: 233. Dar al-Kitab: Cairo.

22 Lee E (1985) Asian infant feeding. *Nursing Mirror*; **160**: S14–15.

23 Black J (1985) Asian families II – conditions that may be found in children. *BMJ*; **290**: 830–3.

24 Aukett A, Wharton B (1989) Nutrition of Asian children. In: JK Cruickshanks, DG Beevers (eds) *Ethnic Factors in Health and Disease*, pp. 241–8. Butterworth-Heinemann: Oxford.

25 Harries RJ, Armstrong D, Ali R, Loynes A (1983) Nutritional survey of Bangladeshi children aged under 5 years in the London Borough of Tower Hamlets. *Arch Dis Child*; **58**: 428–32.

26 Oppe TE, Arneil GC, Davies DP *et al.* (1980) *Present Day Practice in Infant Feeding: report of a Working Party of the Panel on Child Nutrition, Committee on Medical Aspects of Food Policy (Reports on health and social subjects; 20)*, p. 21. HMSO: London.

27 Gatrad AR (1984) *The Muslim in Hospital, School and the Community* (PhD thesis). University of Wolverhampton.

28 Ali YA (1938) *The Meaning of the Glorious Quran*; **7**: 157 (trans modified). Dar al-Kitab: Cairo.

29 El-Hashemite N (1997) The Islamic view in genetic preventive procedures. *Lancet*; **350**: 223.

30 Salihu HM (1997) Genetic counselling among Muslims: questions remain unanswered. *Lancet*; **350**: 1035.

31 Al-Qaradawi Y (1960) *The Lawful and the Prohibited in Islam*, pp. 222–7. ATP: Indianapolis.

CHAPTER 7

Managing the fasting patient: sacred ritual, modern challenges

(★ *Ahmed Sadiq*

The practice of fasting has a long and rich history – it has been used famously to political effect by Mahatma Gandhi, as part of slimming fads, particularly in the West, and also for medicinal reasons such as the pre-operative fast. Above all, though it remains an important religious ritual for many of the major faith groups, notable examples of which include the Yom Kippur fast of Judaism and the Lent fast still observed by some Eastern Christian sects. The Muslim fast of Ramadan, involving over one in six of all humans, is however the most widely observed celebration of this most sacred of rituals; hence healthcare professionals are very likely to come into most intimate contact with fasting when caring for Muslims.[1] After briefly discussing the meaning of the Muslim fast, I consider the rules and regulations governing fasting, using this as a basis to explore the implications of fasting for health and healthcare provision. The chapter concludes with the presentation of four case histories illustrating some of the central issues discussed.

The fast of Ramadan
A blessed month
The month of Ramadan, the ninth of the Islamic calendar, is distinguished above all others because it was during this month, over 14 centuries ago, that the revelation of the Qur'an began. Allah had, in His wisdom and mercy, chosen Muhammad as His final Emissary, responsible for communicating the Divine Word to 'all the Worlds'. Ramadan thus marks the unfolding of a familiar but

distinct chapter in religious history; familiar in that the message is a reaffirmation and re-articulation of that delivered by Abraham, Moses, David, John the Baptist and Christ, distinct for this marked Allah's final reminder.

There is an entire literature devoted to the merits of Ramadan, encouraging and exhorting the believers to 'free' themselves from the grip of 'this world'; Muhammad taught that not only are good acts magnified innumerably during the month, but a gate of Paradise is dedicated to the fasting. For the man and the woman in the street then, Ramadan is synonymous with blessing; the flurry of activity through telephone lines that follow the sighting of the new moon, carrying the simple but telling message '*Mubarak*', 'congratulations' – in that you are fortunate enough to once again partake of its blessings – bears testimony to the importance of Ramadan in the Muslim psyche. The sense of loss that marks the end of the month is real and tangible.

Preparing for Ramadan

'You should work only for the hereafter in this noble month, and embark on something worldly only when absolutely necessary. Arrange your life before Ramadan in a manner that will render you free for worship when it arrives. Be intent on devotions and approach Allah more surely, especially during the last ten days.'

– Abdallah ibn Alawi Al-Hadad[2]

The meaning of fasting

Within Muslim ethic fasting is above all a spiritual exercise, serving a range of diverse but complementary functions (Table 7.1). Its central aim is to afford an opportunity to reflect on one's relationships – both with Allah and with one's fellow man. A customary greeting of Muslims is to greet friends and relatives by saying, 'If I have wronged you, please forgive me.'[3] The sense of solidarity engendered by such collective devotion helps to locate the believer temporally and geographically in the fraternity of faith.

TABLE 7.1 Why Muslims fast

Fasting:
- Teaches the principle of sincerity as a Muslim fasts to please Allah alone.
- Cultivates a consciousness of the Divine because a fasting person keeps his fast without any human authority checking his actions.
- Develops empathy with the less fortunate through sharing temporarily in their pain and hunger.
- Teaches moderation, willpower, self-reassurance, self-control and self-discipline.
- Inculcates a spirit of social belonging, unity, brotherhood and equality as it joins together a whole Muslim society in observing the same sacred ritual, in the same manner, at the same time, for the same reasons, throughout the world.

The rules of fasting

A fasting Muslim abstains from all food, drink and intimate relations from dawn to sunset. This is a total and complete abstinence. Smoking also breaks the fast.

The fast is not nullified if one, through forgetfulness, inadvertently transgress these rules, so long as the act in question is ceased as soon as one realises one's error. There are no restrictions on consuming lawful food and drink between sunset and dawn, but it is considered distasteful to overeat since one of the central aims of fasting is to learn self-control. This self-control needs to extend beyond the material into the realm of social relationships and it is required that the fasting person should also avoid lying, backbiting and engaging in frivolous or obscene conversation.[4] These values should of course continue throughout the remainder of the year.

The Islamic calendar is lunar (about nine to 10 days shorter than the solar year); therefore, during the course of a lifetime, Ramadan will fall during all four seasons. In Britain, for example, a winter fast lasts on average for 10 hours; in contrast, a summer fast may be for almost 19 hours. For those who live in extreme latitudes, where there may be total darkness or total daylight for months continuously, Islamic Law is flexible in its application, requiring fasting for the length of time being fasted in a neighbouring region where the normal cycle of day and night is preserved.[5]

Fasting is obligatory on every responsible and healthy Muslim, male and female. Table 7.2 details those exempt from fasting. If a fast is missed intentionally, without valid excuse, then the penalty for each missed day is to fast consecutively for two months or to provide a meal for 60 people. Otherwise, the expiation is to fast one day for each missed or nullified fast.

TABLE 7.2 Those exempt from fasting

- Children under the age of puberty.*
- Those with learning difficulties or retardation such that they are unable to comprehend the nature and purpose of the fast.*
- The old and frail who are not capable of fasting.[†]
- The acutely unwell for whom fasting will exacerbate their condition.[‡]
- Those with chronic illnesses, in whom fasting may be detrimental to health.[‡]
- Travellers (who are journeying greater than approximately 50 miles) if they feel they may be harmed by the fast.[‡]
- Menstruating women.[‡]
- Pregnant and nursing women if they fear for their own health, or that of their children.[‡]

Notes: *atonement not required; [†]should feed a destitute person for every missed day; [‡]the missed fasts are required to be made up one day for each day missed when the reason for exemption has expired.

Fasting and health

Medical exemptions

During sickness, the exemption from fasting may be temporary or permanent. Temporary exemption may be exercised by those patients who have an acute illness where fasting may aggravate their illness and delay recovery; for example, those with renal colic whose condition may be aggravated by dehydration, or those requiring antibiotics for an infective episode. Once in good health, the patient should make up for the missed fasts at a later date. A permanent exemption may be applied to the elderly and frail, or those with certain intractable conditions such as systemic cancer, who will therefore not be in a position to make up missed fasts in the future. The chronically ill may substitute their fasting by providing food for the poor.

Islam encourages the maintenance of good health, even at the expense of fasting during Ramadan. In cases where patients are unsure whether it is appropriate to fast due to health considerations, they are encouraged to seek a medical opinion. In cases of uncertainty, a doctor's decision as to whether fasting, or the inability to take medication in the daylight hours, would be deleterious to a patient's health is totally acceptable and should be adhered to (SM Darsh, personal communication, 1995). However, evidence seems to suggest that some patients do not approach their family practitioners in this regard.[1] They may feel that a non-Muslim physician is very likely to prohibit fasting (even when there are no associated health risks) on account of a failure to understand the significance and importance of fasting. In such cases, many choose to adjust their own medication timings to fit in with the times when eating is allowed.

A study which looked at the drug regimens of 81 patients during Ramadan found that 46% changed their drug dosage pattern while fasting.[6] This consisted of missing doses, altering the timing of doses, or taking all the day's medications at one time. In many cases this is perhaps of little consequence, but as discussed in the case histories that follow, such practice can at times have serious consequences. For example, unless taken following medical advice, short-acting agents may lose their effect some time into the fast. In addition, a larger dose taken once daily may have toxic side effects, especially in the elderly. As a rule, it would be far better for patients to discuss medication changes with clinicians in advance of any planned change; this does, however, require clinicians and pharmacists to have an appreciation of Muslim teaching regarding the importance of fasting, the use of medication while fasting, and also an understanding of the metabolic effects of controlled fasting.

Medication use

Allowing anything to enter through the mouth into the intestine nullifies the fast,[5] therefore any medication that is swallowed will also invalidate the fast. For those who require oral medication, dosage times can usually be easily and safely altered so that tablets are taken before the start and at the end of the fast, or in some cases by switching from short-acting agents to longer-acting ones. Such an approach is particularly convenient for oral treatments for many gastrointestinal, cardiovascular, respiratory, central nervous system, endocrine and rheumatic disorders, as well as for nutritional supplements.

If there is a necessity for the medication during the daytime, for example to preserve life, then the person is considered to be sick and has the dispensation not to fast as discussed previously. For those in whom such a situation arises while fasting, there is no harm whatsoever in abandoning the fast since heroic acts of misplaced piety have nothing to do with the teachings of Islam.

If a medication is not swallowed but enters into the body or bloodstream, and it is not a source of nutrition, it does not invalidate the fast. This means that while fasting, medication may be taken by all routes except orally. Hence patients are able to take sublingual medication such as nitrates for angina, since these are neither swallowed (but are rapidly absorbed into the bloodstream) nor are they nutritious. This is unlike a substance such as sugar, which, even when placed under the tongue, dissolves in saliva and is then swallowed rather than absorbed by the sublingual blood vessels.

The use of parenteral fluids or nutrition is prohibited while fasting as this involves the use of procedures designed to bypass the alimentary tract, thus having important systemic effects and also being of nutritional value. Injection of non-nutritious agents, such as local anaesthetics, is allowed. Agents that primarily have a topical mode of action, such as eye drops, are, however, acceptable since jurists have ruled that 'the eye is not one of the apertures leading to the stomach'. Although eye drops are not swallowed, small amounts may be absorbed systemically from the conjunctiva and nasal mucosa. Patients who still have reservations, despite adequate explanation, could be encouraged to perform lachrymal punctual occlusion following drop insertion as this will reduce the amount of the fluid entering the nose. Skin-patch delivery systems, for example nitrates for angina, can be used while fasting, as again the medication is not swallowed, but is rapidly absorbed into the bloodstream. Nevertheless, skin patches delivering nicotine should not be used as the use of nicotine, in whatever form, is not in keeping with the spirit of the fast. Skin creams and other topical medications are also allowed for similar reasons. The withdrawing of blood for testing and donation is allowed.

While all agree that the use of oral medications (syrups, tablets, capsules) is prohibited during fasting, the use of other types of medication while fasting is a more contentious area. Most jurists are of the opinion that the use of inhalers for asthma is allowed, but should only be used if needed (as there is a risk that part of the 'inhaled' medication may enter the oesophagus). Treatment could be tailored with the use of long-acting inhalers and/or slow release oral medication when not fasting. Nose and ear drops are not allowed unless absolutely needed, and then should not enter the throat. Use of per rectal and per urethral medication is not allowed while fasting.

These principles are similarly applied to dental procedures. Mouthwashes and toothpaste are allowed, but their use is considered to be highly undesirable as the deliberate or accidental swallowing of them will nullify the fast. This is because the risk of swallowing is known beforehand to be high. The use of *miswaak* (a stick used to clean the teeth) is highly recommended at all times, including while fasting. This is a form of oral hygiene commonly used in Muslim countries with many beneficial properties. The use of varnishes, pulp-capping medicaments and the placement of antibiotics in the mouth is similarly allowed. Anti-fungals in the form of pastilles or lozenges can only be used outside fasting hours. As the working site is in the mouth, many patients with non-urgent problems prefer to be seen and treated either after sunset or after Ramadan has ended. Patients who are ill or in acute discomfort have a temporary exemption from fasting for medical reasons as discussed above.

Faced with the fasting patient, it is important for professionals to be aware of which treatments the *individual* considers acceptable, and offer treatment accordingly. Though the principles outlined above are shared by all, individual interpretations can and do vary.[7] This should come as no great surprise since many of the treatment modalities discussed had no precedence at the time of the Prophet; in such circumstances Islamic Law requires jurists to consider the issues, using the principles enshrined in the primary sources of law and arrive at a decision. That jurists may initially come to differing conclusions is expected and indeed welcome (*see* Chapter 4) – in many cases a consensus opinion evolves with the passage of time.

Implications for health

Most scientific studies investigating the effects of fasting during Ramadan have been performed in Muslim countries. Some of the results may therefore not be directly applicable to Muslims living in temperate areas, where the risk of dehydration is significantly lower than for those living in the equatorial regions of Asia and the Arabian peninsula, for example. Because of the dearth of local research, extrapolation from available data is made wherever this is considered reasonable. It is also important to be aware that much of Western research on the subject has focused on the ill-effects of fasting; in view of the tensions that exist between religion and science in post-Enlightenment Europe this is perhaps not surprising.

Ramadan entails a significant change to the daily routine, with many choosing to spend long periods of the night awake. Modification of the wake/sleep cycle causes an alteration in bodily circadian rhythm for a month; this returns to normal at the end of Ramadan. Meals are taken during the night hours and extra time is spent in prayers and worship, resulting in sleep being delayed and quite considerably shorter than outside Ramadan, especially when the period falls during the longer summer months. Some may catch up with lost sleep during the afternoon or early evening, but this is often not possible for those in full-time employment. This can result in a gradual increase in tiredness and mild sleep deprivation as the month continues. The physical features of fatigue and exhaustion produced by fasting have been shown objectively to reduce cognitive function in some people, as measured by reduced visual flicker fusion.[8]

In the healthy, normal homeostatic mechanisms ensure that controlled fasting has little effect on body biochemistry. Hypoglycaemia is thus not an issue in non-diabetics, for example. In the hot summer days, the prohibition of fluids may lead to mild dehydration, resulting in the common symptoms of dizziness, nausea and headaches, accompanied with a resting tachycardia. The risks of dehydration while fasting may be exaggerated, as shown by a study by Abdalla and colleagues investigating the effects of fasting on those who are over one year post-renal transplantation – no impairment in graft function was observed.[9]

There appears to be no significant overall change in body weight during the month.[10] Exceptions may of course occur, and fluid loss may be responsible for any initial weight loss seen in some people,[11] while paradoxically the weight of some people may increase a little during the month. An increased consumption of high-calorific fried foods when opening the fast – common among some – seems the most plausible explanation. Thirst is felt more intensely than hunger, and one tends to feel the cold more, especially when fasting long hours, a consequence of a slowing down of the body's metabolic rate in order to conserve energy stores.[11]

Though changes in serum lipids are variable, there appears to be an overall beneficial effect on serum apolipoprotein metabolism.[12] Changes in meal times also change the normal circadian rhythm for intragastric acidity,[13] resulting in an increase in acid and pepsin secretion,[14] and this appears to be the likely basis for the observed increased risk of peptic ulcer complications during Ramadan.[15] Particular care therefore needs to be taken when advising patients with a history of peptic ulcer disease about the risks associated with fasting.

Although expectant and nursing mothers can be exempt from fasting (Table 7.2), many choose to fast (AR Gatrad, personal communication, 1999). Their reasons are simple, and include a combination of preferring to fast with their families rather than make up the time later when they may be fasting alone and a reverence for the blessings associated with fasting in the holy month. Interestingly, fasting during Ramadan has been shown not to affect the mean birth weight of babies at any stage of pregnancy.[16] Mothers may report that their babies move very little during daylight hours, but this is compensated for by increased activity at night. This is because the diurnal cycle of the foetus changes with that of its mother. Fasting does tend to change the concentrations of lactose, sodium and potassium in breast milk, but the quantity of milk only tends to change during long fasts or fasts in hot countries, due to maternal dehydration.

Although harder to quantify than physical changes, Ramadan appears to have a beneficial effect on psychological well-being. Little research in this area exists, but a study of British university students showed that an increased proportion became involved in spiritual and other stress-reducing activities during Ramadan.[17] Another study has found that significantly fewer parasuicides were reported during Ramadan than at other times.[18] Although this particular study was performed in Jordan, it seems reasonable to conclude that one may expect a similar or an even greater effect in the West because of the relatively limited stabilising and protective effect of family cohesiveness in migrant Muslim populations when compared with native Muslim communities. This protective effect of Ramadan may, to the Muslim mind, be explained by the blessings inherent in the month itself, in addition to the more common sociological interpretation of increased family and communal solidarity associated with a common sense of purpose.

Of all research into fasting, that into diabetes is most well developed. Despite the theoretical hazards of fasting in patients with diabetes, in practice few complications occur.[19–21] In fact, fasting may even prove beneficial through weight loss and decreased food intake.[20,21] Table 7.3 summarises current advice for diabetics while fasting.[22] Patients should, however, consult their diabetic practitioner for individual advice.

TABLE 7.3 Summary of recommendations for diabetic patients wishing to fast[22]

Diet-controlled
- Make the pre-dawn meal the major meal of the day.
- Space meals equally over the non-fasting period.

On oral hypoglycaemic agents
- If on a single daily dose, take medication with the sunset meal.
- For those on more than a once-daily regimen switch the morning dose (plus any midday dose) with that taken at sunset.

On insulin
- Fasting is not recommended in those prone to keto-acidosis or with wide swings in blood glucose.
- If on a single daily dose, change to a twice-daily regimen.
- For those on a twice-daily regimen, take half or one-third of the morning insulin dose and take the usual evening dose.
- Those taking basal bolus insulin should split the long-acting (basal) component into two equal doses taken during the sunset and pre-dawn meals, and take the rapid acting (bolus) component as previously, but omitting the middle dose.

Organisational considerations
The epidemiology of fasting

The overwhelming majority of Muslims choose to fast during Ramadan. Gatrad has, for example, shown that over 90% of adult Muslims in Walsall, England fast, and there is no reason to believe that this figure is any different in other Muslim communities.[23] In view of such high proportions fasting, it seems reasonable to assume, when considering organisational issues, that Muslims are fasting. Needless to say, when dealing with individual patients it is far better to ask about individual practices and preferences, rather than assume.

Hospital attendance

Time, considered a sacred commodity in classical Islamic understanding, is of a premium during Ramadan. The poor outpatient attendance by Muslims during the month is thus hardly surprising as non-urgent matters are typically delayed until after Ramadan.[24] In consequence, there may be a small increased demand for acute service provision, reflected in the increased use of accident and emergency departments noted in at least one study.[25] These casualty visits tend to be late at night as patients do not want to receive interventions or treatments that may invalidate their fast.

More interesting, however, is that with appropriate planning and consideration of religious sensitivities it is possible to dramatically improve outpatient attendance rates. Using a complex intervention involving, among other things, the use of multicultural calendars by clinic staff,[26] thereby allowing staff to avoid important religious festivals such as Ramadan, Gatrad has shown that it is possible to reduce the proportion of patients failing to attend paediatric outpatient appointments from 50% to 12% over a three year period.[27]

Primary care

For those working in areas with large Muslim populations, it seems important that general practitioners, nurses and community pharmacists receive some training with respect to managing the fasting patient. As far as I am aware no such provision currently exists. Many Jewish and Hindu patients will also fast at particular times during the year,[1] although the nature of the fast in these traditions is not necessarily identical to the Muslim fast. Such a training programme could also tackle issues and concerns raised by members of these communities. In particular, it would seem prudent to encourage patients to consult their primary care staff well in advance of Ramadan to discuss issues regarding the safety of fasting and any possible medication changes. This may be important for patients who suffer from chronic conditions such as diabetes, asthma, epilepsy, hypertension and psychiatric illnesses. The patient would require review just before Ramadan to ensure good health prior to fasting, and just after Ramadan so that they can either return to their previous regimen or continue with their new regimen if this proved to be preferable or more efficacious.[28,29]

Case studies

Case 1: epilepsy

A patient was admitted to hospital having had a seizure while driving. Prior to this episode his epilepsy had been well controlled on phenytoin 100 mg three times daily. Observing the fast of Ramadan, which had commenced only three days earlier, he had omitted his morning and afternoon doses, on each of the three days.

Comment

Failing to understand the nature of the Ramadan fast, he was labelled as 'non-compliant' by the hospital staff. Because of the long half-life of phenytoin, he could quite easily have been changed to phenytoin 300 mg taken as a single daily dose. Such a change should ideally have taken place before the start of Ramadan.

Case 2: glaucoma

A middle-aged woman suffering from glaucoma had been prescribed eye drops to be used four times daily at regular intervals. During Ramadan, she wished to fast and so decided to use her eye drops only during the night; in practice this involved instilling the drops only once daily. During the course of the month her glaucoma deteriorated.

Comment

She could easily have continued taking her eye drops during Ramadan as eye drops do not invalidate the fast. Being unaware, without the safety net of pro-active, structured care provision, she lost her vision unnecessarily.

Case 3: chronic rheumatoid arthritis

A 54-year-old South Asian man with chronic rheumatoid arthritis, well controlled on daily non-steroidal anti-inflammatory medication, consulted his general practitioner to discuss alternative treatment options for the forthcoming Ramadan period. His GP thought it best to switch to suppositories. The patient failed to use the suppositories as inserting medication rectally would have nullified his fast. This resulted in an increase in pain and stiffness.

Comment

Apart from nullifying the fast for Muslims, there is a strong stigma against the use of medication per rectum in many cultures. A more appropriate choice with this patient may have been to switch to a long-acting oral preparation taken once daily with his largest meal. If found to be well controlled at the post-Ramadan review, there would be no harm in his continuing with this treatment regimen beyond Ramadan.

Case 4: psychiatry

A woman suffering from depression and other psychiatric problems was prescribed a combination of antidepressants and neuroleptics. During Ramadan she insisted on fasting despite the fact that she had reason for exemption on medical grounds and was informed of this by family members. Concerned that a failure to comply with medication might result in deterioration in her mental state, the family took advice from a Muslim scholar who was held in high regard by the patient. The scholar advised the patient that she was permitted to continue her medication while 'fasting'. His advice was heeded.

Comment

This woman was quite rightly advised not to fast as she was exempt due to her psychiatric illness with a very real possibility of her mental state deteriorating if compliance was poor. She insisted on fasting, but was persuaded that taking the medication would not invalidate her fast, which of course it does!

Summary

➥ While fasting is common to many religious and cultural traditions, healthcare professionals are likely to come into most intimate contact with fasting when caring for Muslim patients. The overwhelming majority of Muslims observe the fast of Ramadan.

➥ In the event of a fast posing health risks, Muslims are exempt from fasting. In cases where individuals are unsure of the possible health risks, Islamic Law recommends that the advice of a medical practitioner be sought.

➥ The use of oral medication is prohibited while fasting. However, it is possible, in most cases, to alter preparations and dosage times easily and safely, so that medication need only be taken outside of daylight hours. Medications that are neither swallowed nor of nutritious value do not invalidate the fast.

➥ Time is considered particularly precious during Ramadan, explaining why a large proportion of Muslims choose not to attend clinic and outpatient appointments during the holy months. Incorporating a multicultural calendar into the appointment-booking template should allow important religious festivals to be more easily recognised by clinic staff, thereby allowing an alternative appointment to be offered.

Acknowledgements

I wish to thank Dr M Aslam PhD, Head of Clinical Pharmacy, University of Nottingham, for allowing the case studies to be reproduced. Table 7.3 is adapted, with permission, from a paper in the *Journal of the Royal Society of Medicine*. Finally, I thank the reviewers and editors for their constructive criticism on earlier drafts of this chapter.

References

1 Sadiq SA, Sheikh A (1999) The fasting patient. *Update*, **59**: 639–45.
2 al-Haddad AI (1989) *The Book of Assistance*, p. 71. Quilliam Press: London.
3 Waddy C (1976) *The Muslim Mind*, p. 9. Longman: London.
4 Abdalati H (1975) *Islam in Focus*, p. 210. IPCI: Birmingham.

5 Sabiq AS (1991) *Fiqh us-Sunnah*, vol III, p. 166. American Trust Publications: Washington.

6 Aslam M, Healy M (1986) Compliance and drug therapy in fasting Moslem patients. *J Clin Hosp Pharm*; **11**: 321–5.

7 Sheikh A (1998) Medical implications of controlled fasting. *J R Soc Med*; **91**: 453.

8 Ali M, Amir T (1989) Effects of fasting on visual flicker fusion. *Percept Motor Skills*; **69**: 627–31.

9 Abdalla AH, Shaheen FA, Rassoul Z, *et al.* (1998) Effect of Ramadan fasting on Moslem kidney transplant recipients. *Am J Nephrol*; **18**: 101–4.

10 Finch GM, Day JE, Razak, Welch DA, Rogers PJ (1998) Appetite changes under free-living conditions during Ramadan. *Appetite*; **31**: 159–70.

11 Sweileh N, Schnitzler A, Hunter GR, Davis B (1992) Body composition and energy metabolism in resting and exercising Muslims during Ramadan fast. *J Sport Med Physical Fitness*; **32**: 156–63.

12 Adlouni A, Ghalim N, Saile R, Hda N, Parra HJ, Benslimane A (1998) Beneficial effect on serum apo AI, apo B and Lp AI levels of Ramadan fasting. *Clin Chem Acta*; **271**: 179–89.

13 Lanzon-Miller S, Pounder R (1991) The effect of fasting on 24-hour intragastric acidity and plasma gastrin. *Am J Gastro*; **86**: 165–7.

14 Hakkou F, Tazi A, Iraqui L, Celice-Pingaud C, Vatier J (1994) The observance of Ramadan and its repercussion on gastric secretion. *Gastro Clin Biol*; **18**: 190–4.

15 Donderici O, Temizhan A, Kucukbas T, Eskioglu E (1994) Effect of Ramadan on peptic ulcer complications. *Scand J Gastro*; **29**: 603–6.

16 Cross JH, Eminson J, Wharton BA (1990) Ramadan and birth weight at full term in Asian Moslem pregnant women in Birmingham. *Arch Dis Child*; **65**: 1053–6.

17 Afifi ZE (1997) Daily practices, study performance and health during the Ramadan fast. *J R Soc Hlth*; **117**: 231–5.

18 Daradkeh T (1992) Parasuicide during Ramadan in Jordan. *Acta Psych Scand*; **86**: 253–4.

19 Belkhadir J, Ghomari H, Klocker N, Mikou A, Nasciri M, Sabri M (1993) Muslims with non-insulin dependent diabetes fasting during Ramadan: treatment with glibenclamide. *BMJ*; **307**: 292–5.

20 Lajaam M (1990) Ramadan fasting and non-insulin dependent diabetes: effect on metabolic control. *East Afr Med J*; **67**: 732–6.

21 Mafauzy M, Mohammed W, Anum M, Zulkifli A, Ruhani A (1990) A study of the fasting diabetic patients during the month of Ramadan. *Med J Malay*; **45**: 14–17.

22 Fazel M (1998) Medical implications of controlled fasting. *J R Soc Med*; **91**: 260–3.

23 Gatrad AR (1994) *The Muslim in Hospital, School and the Community* (PhD thesis). University of Wolverhampton.

24 Gatrad AR (1997) Comparison of Asian and English non-attenders at a hospital outpatient department. *Arch Dis Child*; **77**: 423–6.

25 Langford E, Ishaque M, Fothergill J, Touquet R (1994) The effect of Ramadan on accident and emergency attendances. *J R Soc Med*; **87**: 517–8.

26 Gould C, Rose D, Woodward P (eds) (1999) *SHAP Calendar of Religious Festivals*. SHAP Working Party: London.

27 Gatrad AR (2000) A completed audit to reduce hospital outpatient non-attendance rates. *Arch Dis Child*; **82**: 59–61.

28 Car J, Sheikh A (2004) Fasting and asthma: an opportunity for building patient-doctor partnership. *Prim Care Respir J*; **13**: 133–5.

29 Sheikh A (2007) Should Muslims have faith based health services? *BMJ*; **334**: 74.

CHAPTER 8

Hajj: journey of a lifetime

☪ *Abdul Rashid Gatrad and Aziz Sheikh*

Ever since childhood, five times a day, many a Muslim will have turned his whole being in prayer towards The Sacred Mosque in Mecca, Saudi Arabia. Journeying to Mecca for Hajj (pilgrimage) is therefore no ordinary undertaking. For many, Hajj represents the culmination of years of spiritual preparation and planning. Once completed the pilgrim is given the honorific title *Hajji* (pilgrim).

Hajj commemorates the Patriarch Abraham's readiness to sacrifice his son Ishmael in biblical times. Performing Hajj is one of the five pillars of Islam and is therefore obligatory for all adult Muslims who can afford to undertake the journey and are in good health. Hajj lasts for five days and as the Islamic calendar is lunar, the precise Gregorian calendar dates will vary each year by about 10 days. Muslims travel to Mecca at other times to perform a lesser pilgrimage called *Umrah*.

Mecca has a resident population of about 200 000, this swelling to well over two million during the Hajj season. This rapid increase in numbers poses many challenges, including ensuring adequate food, water and sanitary facilities both in Mecca and the neighbouring deserts of Mina and Arafat, which pilgrims must visit as part of the Hajj ritual.

Although only incumbent on a Muslim once in a lifetime, many, and in particular those residing in the West, will journey far more frequently. For example, over 20 000 Britons perform the Hajj each year and the current annual figure for Umrah stands at almost 29 000.[1] In view of the very large numbers of people from disparate regions and the hostile climate of the Arabian Desert, the chance of disease striking, particularly the elderly and the infirm, is high.

In this chapter, we briefly describe the main rites of the Hajj before focusing on particular health risks associated with the Hajj and measures that may be taken to minimise such risks.

The significance of Hajj

The Sacred Mosque (Ka'bah)

'A curious object, that Ka'bah! There it stands at this hour, in the black cloth-covering the Sultan sends it yearly; 'twenty-seven cubits high'; with circuit, with double circuit of pillars, with festoon-rows of lamps and quaint ornaments: the lamps will be lighted again this night – to glitter again under the stars. An authentic fragment of the oldest Past. It is the Qiblah (direction of prayer) of all Muslims: from Delhi all onwards to Morocco, the eyes of innumerable praying men are turned towards it, five times, this day and all days: one of the notablest centres in the Habitation of Men.'

– Thomas Carlyle[2]

According to Muslim tradition, The Sacred Mosque was the first temple erected for the worship of Allah. It stands then as a symbol of monotheism. Many of the rites of the Hajj date back to the Prophet Abraham, one of the outstanding figures in Muslim history. Mecca is also honoured because it is the birthplace of Muhammad, Allah's final Messenger to Man. In common with pilgrimages in other faiths, the Hajj is a deeply spiritual exercise; a journey of heightened self-consciousness and individual self-renewal.

Journeying home

'And when, as a pilgrim, he stands before the Ka'bah in Mecca (after circling it seven times), the centrality already prefigured by his orientation when he prayed far off is made actual. Clothed only in two pieces of plain, unsewn cloth, he has left behind him the characteristics which identified him in the world, his race, his nationality, his status; he is no longer so-and-so from such-and-such a place, but simply a pilgrim.

'Beneath his bare feet, like mother-of-pearl, is the pale marble of this amphitheatre at the centre of the world, and although he is commanded to lower his eyes when praying elsewhere, he is now permitted to raise them and look upon the Ka'bah, which is the earthly shadow of the Pole or Pivot around which circle the starry heavens. Although Paradise may still seem far distant, he has already come home.'

– Gai Eaton[3]

The rites of Hajj

Many prospective pilgrims fail to appreciate that Hajj is physically demanding. It is the most complex of the Islamic rituals and involves, among other things, walking long distances and camping in desert tents, often with only the most basic sanitation.[4] Centrepiece in these activities is the pilgrim's presence on the desert plain of Arafah, from noon until sundown. Here, dressed in the simplest possible garb made up of two pieces of unstitched cloth for men (*Ihram*), with women wearing their usual clothing, with a head scarf, pilgrims will spend much of the day standing in humility and prayer, performing a dress rehearsal for the final standing before God on Judgement Day.

Because of the sheer volume of human traffic, performing even the simplest rites can take an extraordinary length of time. There is a religious dispensation for those in poor health and many will make use of this allowance after consultation with their doctor;[5] some will, however, travel against medical advice, often in the hope of dying in the Holy Land. For Muslims living in the West the decision of whether or not to travel on health grounds is often more complex since few health professionals have an awareness of what the Hajj entails and its associated health risks, and therefore typically find it difficult to offer an informed opinion.

Health problems and approaches to minimising risks
Problems of sun and heat

Next please!

'In the next few days prostration from (heat) exposure passed at a rapid clip through the hotel. Striking down groups of four or five, it moved from room to room and floor to floor. Soon the hotel began to resemble an infirmary, with dozens of guests in various stages of illness strewn around the lobby every night. Guides were not spared.

'Every day the temperature climbed by one or two degrees. At midnight the mercury remained above one hundred Fahrenheit . . .'

– Michael Wolfe[6]

Travelling to Mecca in advance of the Hajj is sensible, particularly for those unaccustomed to the oppressive climate of the Arab Desert. Pilgrims need to be made aware that acclimatisation – which occurs through a gradual increase in sweat production thereby facilitating cooling through increased water evaporation – to very high temperatures can take between one and two weeks.[7]

Sunburn is a significant hazard, particularly for the light-skinned. The use of an appropriate strength sun block is important to minimise the risks of burning, with its associated risk of malignant tumours. More importantly, it is crucial that sun exposure is kept to a minimum as discussed below.

Heat exhaustion and heat stroke are common, and can be fatal. The Saudi authorities, in their role as the pilgrims' hosts, undertake valuable health promotional work, distributing leaflets and issuing radio and television warnings of the dangers of excessive sun exposure. The number of people who still succumb to the heat is, however, evidence enough that the message needs to be reiterated at every possible opportunity.[8]

During the Hajj men are prohibited from directly covering their heads (with a hat or scarf, for example), thereby increasing the risk of significant heat exposure. The usefulness of a quality umbrella, preferably white in colour, so as to reflect away the sun's rays, cannot be overemphasised. Such simple measures may be life-saving if the pilgrim were to lose his or her bearing in the desert, as is easily and not infrequently done. Other important precautionary measures that may be taken are summarised in Table 8.1.

TABLE 8.1 Precautionary measures to minimise the risk of heat exhaustion and heat stroke

- Avoid spending long periods of time in the sun, particularly when it is at its zenith.
- Travel by night whenever possible (which may also avoid stampedes).
- Keep heads covered during the day (with an umbrella if necessary).
- Consume large volumes of fluid throughout the day.
- Always keep a canister of fluid in your possession.
- Increase dietary salt intake or use salt tablets.
- Avoid transport in 'open top' buses.

Heat exhaustion typically occurs in subjects who are not acclimatised and undertake strenuous exercise. Water depletion or a combination of salt and water depletion, due to excessive sweating, is the underlying cause. Water loss can be as much as five litres per day, and up to 20 grams of salt may be lost. Most cases are relatively mild, with symptoms of weakness, light-headedness and muscle cramps that will respond to a combination of rest, cooling, fluid and salt replacement. If not adequately treated, however, heat stroke may occur.[7,9]

Heat stroke is a medical emergency (Table 8.2; and *see* Table 8.3 for emergency contact numbers). Skin is hot to the touch and there is a notable absence of sweating. The very young, the elderly and diabetics are most at risk. The extreme rise in body temperature makes prompt and appropriate treatment mandatory. The patient should be moved into the shade, stripped, cooled with a combination of fanning and spraying the body with cold water, and, if conscious, given fluid replacement, while expert medical attention is urgently sought.

TABLE 8.2 Symptoms suggestive of heat exhaustion and heat stroke

- Fatigue, weakness and leg cramps.
- Headache, nausea and vomiting.
- Giddiness.
- Delirium.
- Syncope and coma.

TABLE 8.3 Emergency numbers in Saudia Arabia

Ambulance	997
Police	999

Since the early 1980s, cooling units have been installed along the pilgrim route. Emergency services will often suspend patients in a hammock-like bed and spray them liberally with an air/water mixture. The water is warm and cools the body through evaporation, simultaneously also preventing further dehydration. Research suggests that these simple devices are significantly quicker in reducing body temperature than the usual method of placing victims in an ice bath. This is possibly explained by the fact that unlike with the ice bath method, vasoconstriction and shivering are not induced – responses which ultimately cause the body temperature to rise.[10]

Most pilgrims travel on foot; quality footwear is important, though in our experience, frequently overlooked. During the day, the desert sand typically becomes burning hot. Care needs to be taken to avoid walking barefoot because of the serious risks of foot burns. This is particularly important for diabetics with a neuropathy, as very extensive damage may quickly occur, often compounded by the problems of poor wound healing and the increased risks of infection. Footwear needs to be removed before prayers and those who have not been on Hajj are often unaware of the ease with which footwear can become confused with another pilgrim's and thus inadvertently taken. One may be forced to walk barefoot in an attempt to reclaim one's footwear, with potentially devastating consequences.

Infectious diseases

An outbreak of group A meningococcal meningitis occurred among British Muslim pilgrims following the 1987 Hajj. There were 18 primary cases among pilgrims and 15 subsequent cases among their direct and indirect contacts.[11,12] Similarly, an outbreak of W135 meningococcal disease occurred among British pilgrims in 2000 and 2001. In an attempt to prevent a further outbreak the Saudi authorities now insist that all pilgrims be vaccinated with a single dose of the ACWYVax with conjugate meningitis vaccination.[13] Immunity is thought to last for approximately three years. A medical certificate confirming vaccination is now required before visas will be issued.

Vaccination against hepatitis A and malaria prophylaxis, together with advice on measures to minimise the risk of exposure, are important. We would also recommend vaccination against hepatitis B (*see below*) and influenza, particularly in the context of a possible global influenza pandemic originating from the Hajj.[14] In addition to checking tetanus and polio status, typhoid and diphtheria vaccination should also be considered. Many people decide to travel on from the Hajj, particularly to Africa and the Indian subcontinent, and, therefore, as in all travel consultations, taking a detailed intended travel history is important. Pilgrims need to be reminded of the importance of seeking medical attention for any unexpected symptoms, such as fever, diarrhoea, jaundice or a high fever on their return. A persistent cough is also significant because of the reported high incidence of pneumonia (particularly tuberculous) among pilgrims.[15,16]

One of the rites of the Hajj is for men to have the head shaved (although trimming the hair is also acceptable). Most will have their heads shaved, often in makeshift centres, run by opportunistic 'barbers'. A razor blade is commonly used, and may be used on several scalps before being ultimately discarded. The risks of important blood-borne infections such as HIV and hepatitis B and C are obvious, especially considering that many pilgrims will come from regions of the world where such infections are now endemic.[17] Pilgrims need to be aware of these potential dangers and should insist on the use of a new blade. Physical relationships are prohibited during Hajj, even between husband and wife, and so the risks of acquiring sexually transmitted diseases are minimal.

Injuries

Injuries, particularly to toes, are relatively common, typically resulting from inadvertently being stamped on while barefoot when circumambulating the Ka'bah. More serious injuries, some of which prove to be fatal, occur each year during stampedes in Mina as pilgrims undertake the stoning rite. Pilgrims should be advised to avoid peak times and the old and infirm advised to consider appointing a proxy for the performance of this rite.

General advice

Menstruation is considered a state of ritual impurity, and hence menstruating women are not permitted to perform the Hajj. This often causes a great deal of concern; an emotion that is perfectly understandable if one remembers the importance of the journey and the time, effort and money that may have been invested. Delaying menstrual bleeding, by using the combined oral contraceptive pill or daily progesterone, for example, is perfectly acceptable and many women consult their general practitioners or family planning clinics for this reason in the run up to the Hajj season.

Contact lenses are also often problematic, particularly in arid conditions where sand can often be blown into the eyes. Ocular lubricants (such as Hypromellose 1% eye drops) should be used liberally to stop lenses adhering to the cornea. Temporarily resorting to the use of spectacles may be another option. Although there are a number of makeshift dispensaries erected during the Hajj season, these are often difficult to access, largely on account of the human mass. Pilgrims should therefore ensure that they take enough of their regular medication and small supplies of common remedies, such as analgesia, oral rehydration salts and clove oil for dental pain. A simple travel pack comprising adhesive dressings, an insect repellent, antiseptic cream and water sterilisation tablets is also useful.

Conclusions: the 'Hajj travel consultation'

There are a number of known risks associated with pilgrimage to Mecca which can mar the entire experience. That said, most of these problems should, with sensible precautions, now be preventable. All potential pilgrims must now be protected against meningococcal disease and this opportunity to review patients can be used to impart other key areas of advice discussed above. These issues are summarised in Table 8.4.[18,19]

TABLE 8.4   Issues to consider in the 'Hajj travel consultation'

- Fit to perform the Hajj?
- Heat exhaustion and heat stroke.
- Foot burns and sunburn.
- Infectious diseases.
- General travel advice.

Summary

- Hajj, the journey to The Sacred Mosque in Mecca, is a once-in-a-lifetime obligation for all adult Muslims who are physically and financially able.
- Over two million people globally perform the Hajj each year.
- If unprepared, health risks associated with the Hajj are considerable. Most important are the risks of heat exhaustion, heat stroke and infectious diseases.
- All pilgrims must be vaccinated against meningococcal disease. A 'Hajj travel consultation' is thus mandatory, offering the ideal opportunity for health promotional advice.

References

1 Royal Embassy of Saudi Arabia, London. Press Release, 14 April 1999.
2 Carlyle T (1966) *On Heroes, Hero-worship and the Heroic in History*, pp. 49–50. University of Nebraska Press: Lincoln.
3 Eaton G (1985) *Islam and the Destiny of Man*, p. 242. George Allen and Unwin: London.
4 Sarwar G (1998) *Islam: beliefs and teachings*, pp. 78–81. Muslim Educational Trust: London.
5 Sabiq AS (1992) *Fiqh Us-sunnah: Hajj and umrah*, p. 5. American Trust Publications: Indianapolis.
6 Wolfe M (1994) *The Hadj*, pp. 194–5. Seeker & Warburg: London.
7 Clarke CRA, Clark ML (1994) Environmental medicine. In: PJ Kumar, ML Clark (eds) *Clinical Medicine*, pp. 756–7. Balli're Tindall: London.
8 Seraj ME (1992) Heat stroke during Hajj (pilgrimage) – an update. *Middle East J Anaesthesiol;* **11**: 407–41.
9 Moxham J, Souhami RL, Walker JM. (1990) Physical and environmental causes of disease. In: RL Souhami, J Moxham (eds) *Textbook of Medicine*, pp. 77–8. Longman: London.

10 Henahan J (1982) Treating heat stroke in pilgrims to Mecca. *JAMA*; **247**:3302.

11 Salisbury D, Begg N (eds) (1996) *Immunisation Against Infectious Diseases*, p. 146. The Stationery Office: London.

12 Jones DM, Sutcliffe EM. Group (1990) A meningococcal disease in England associated with the Haj. *J Infect*; **21**: 21–5.

13 Gatrad AR, Shafi S, Memish ZA, Sheikh A (2006) Hajj and the risk of influenza. *BMJ*; **333**: 1182–3.

14 Salisbury D, Begg N (eds) (1996) *Immunisation Against Infectious Diseases*, pp. 147–54. The Stationery Office: London.

15 Alzeer A, Mashlah A, Fakim N *et al.* (1998) Tuberculosis is the commonest cause of pneumonia requiring hospitilization during Hajj. *J Infect*; **36**: 303–6.

16 Yousuf M, Al-Saudi DA, Sheikh RA, Lone MS (1995) Pattern of medical problems among Haj pilgrims admitted King Abdul Aziz Hospital, Madinah Al-Munawarah. *Ann Saudi Med*; **15**: 619–21.

17 Gatrad AR, Sheikh A (2001) Hajj and risk of blood borne infections. *Arch Dis Child*; **84**: 375.

18 Gatrad AR, Sheikh A (2005) Hajj: journey of a lifetime. *BMJ*; **330**: 133–7.

19 Shafi S, Memish ZA, Gatrad AR, Sheikh A (2005) Hajj 2006: communicable disease and other health risks and current official guidance for pilgrims. *Euro Surveill*; **10**: E051215.2.

CHAPTER 9

Death and bereavement: an exploration and a meditation

(★ *Aziz Sheikh and Abdul Rashid Gatrad*

The care of dying patients and their relatives is one of the most difficult aspects of a clinician's job. Enabling an individual to die with dignity can also be deeply rewarding. Providing culturally competent care to the dying requires knowledge and skills – the former in order to minimise the risk of systematic error, the latter in order to apply this information meaningfully to the very *individual* clinical encounter as it unfolds. Sacred Law defines certain expected behaviours at the time of death; our experience, based on witnessing and participating in the deaths of hundreds of our religious affiliates, in many different regions of the world, suggests that these rituals are in the main adhered to by Muslims. Minority Muslim communities often face particular problems in observing certain death customs; these will be highlighted together with a discussion of how these difficulties may impinge on the bereavement process that ensues. The highly topical area of organ donation is considered together with an assessment of how Muslim opinion on this subject is likely to evolve in the years ahead.

Death and dying

> Every soul shall taste death.
>
> – *Qur'an*[1]

Muslim belief regarding death, suicide and euthanasia

For a Muslim, death marks the transition from one state of existence to the next. Islam teaches that life on earth is an examination – the life to come is the eternal abode where one will reap the fruit of one's endeavours on earth (*see* Chapter 2). Death is therefore not to be resisted or fought against, but rather something to be accepted as part of the overall divine plan. Further, death is typically not a taboo subject in Muslim society and is an area that one is encouraged to reflect on frequently.[2] In counselling Muslims regarding a terminal illness or relatives after bereavement, these points should be borne in mind.

Islam views life as sacred and a 'trust' from Allah, thus suicide and deliberate euthanasia are categorically prohibited.[3] Note, however, that undue suffering has no place in Islam and if death is hastened in the process of giving adequate analgesia then this is allowed. What is important is that the primary intent is not to hasten death.

TABLE 9.1 The phases of existence

- Life before conception
- The lower world (life on earth)
- The intermediate realm
- Judgement Day
- The Garden and the Fire

Intent matters

The Prophet (may Allah bless him and grant him peace) said: 'Works are only according to intentions, and a man only receives what he intends.'[4]

The final illness

Considerable distress can be avoided if one is aware of certain death customs that are almost universally practised by Muslims. In keeping with people from most other cultures, ideally Muslims would wish to die at home as making death clinical and remote in a hospital setting is not in keeping with Islamic tradition.[5] The dying person will expect to be visited by friends and relatives, who are encouraged to pray for his or her welfare in the life to come. This is a time when Muslims seek each other's forgiveness for excesses that may have been inadvertently committed. Fifty visitors in the space of a few days would not be exceptional; so strict adherence to the policy of 'two visitors per bed' will cause difficulty for all concerned. Members of the immediate family will often stay by the bedside reciting from the Qur'an, hoping to imbue hope into the heart of a loved one at this most difficult time. Having a copy of the Qur'an on the ward, for those who have not remembered to bring their own, is a kindness. A short passage from the Qur'anic chapter most commonly recited at such times is translated below.

Inspiring hope

The trumpet shall be sounded, when behold! From the sepulchres Man will rush forth to His Lord!

They will say: 'Ah, woe unto us! Who has raised us up from our beds of repose?'

It will be said to them: 'This is what Allah Most Gracious has promised, and true was the word of the apostles!'

It will be no more than a single blast, when lo! They will all be brought before Us! Then, on that Day, not a soul will be wronged in the least, and you shall be repaid for what you used to do.

Verily the companions of the Garden shall that Day have joy in all that they do; they and their spouses will be in groves of cool shade, reclining on thrones of dignity; only delight will there be for them, and theirs shall be all that they could ask for: peace and fulfilment through the word of a Sustainer who dispenses all grace.

– Qur'an[6]

The daily prayers play a pivotal role in the day-to-day life of many a Muslim, and prayer assumes an even greater role in times of suffering and distress. Family members will encourage the dying to continue with their prayers as long as they are able to do so. Before any prayer, ablution is performed; bed-bound patients will need help in this respect. Muslims pray facing Mecca. Again, for the bed-bound, positioning the bed in the direction of Mecca will simplify matters.[7] Recourse to a compass and prayer timetable would be very useful; a prayer timetable is easily available from most local mosques or perhaps more conveniently now from the Internet. Access to a Muslim 'chaplain' may also be helpful, but access to such spiritual care is not always possible.[8,9,10] Many of the visitors and relatives will also need to perform their prayers and it is encouraging to note that hospital prayer facilities are now, in Britain at least, slowly improving.[11,12]

Death rites

When a Muslim dies the eyes and mouth should be closed and the limbs should be straightened. His body should ideally face in the direction of Mecca. It is a religious requirement that the dead be buried as soon as possible and considerable family distress can be avoided by speedy production of the death certificate. The body will be washed and shrouded in simple, unsewn pieces of white cloth – a familiar garb – this having previously been worn as a pilgrim during Hajj while standing on the desert plane of Arafat (*see* Chapter 8). A funeral prayer is held in the local mosque and family and community members follow the funeral procession to the graveyard, where a final prayer is said as the deceased is finally laid to rest, facing towards Mecca. Events occur in rapid succession and in many cases the dead will be buried, particularly in the Muslim countries, within hours of death.[13]

Some turn to Mecca to pray

'We asked the family if they wanted their son's bed facing towards Mecca – they were really taken aback, and so appreciative of such a small gesture!'
                                                                    – Intensive care nurse

---

Accommodating diversity: the British experience

'Two practical questions have arisen for local authorities out of these requirements, namely availability of space in cemeteries allowing the required alignment, and availability of graves at short notice. The solution adopted in most instances has been the allocation of special areas within cemeteries for Muslim burial, a practice which also meets with the community's understandable wish to have Muslims buried in close proximity to each other.'
                                                                    – Jorgen Nielsen[14]

A framework for understanding Muslim bereavement

The subject of Muslim bereavement has received little attention in the biomedical literature.[15] Important questions thus remain with regard to bereavement service provision, particularly since in some quarters it is now argued that primary care staff should provide routine, protocol-driven bereavement care.[16] It is not clear to what degree the various bereavement models currently in vogue are applicable to Muslims, for example, or whether data from cohort studies showing the often-striking association between recent bereavement and subsequent psychological and physical morbidity are applicable to Muslims.[17,18] Our experience suggests that both the above observations appear to have limited face validity with respect to Muslims. Notwithstanding the need for further research, described below is a framework allowing loss and bereavement to be understood from *within* the Muslim tradition. This, we feel, more accurately allows an appreciation of Muslim experiences of bereavement.

Homeward bound

It has already been noted that life has many phases, the hereafter being a palpable reality within the Islamic vision. Within such a framework, the inevitable sense of loss that occurs at the time of death is tempered by the belief that any separation is temporary. Furthermore, there is solace in the knowledge that traversing the bridge of death enables the deceased to re-enter his or her ancestral home, returning to the Highest Company.

A traveller's prayer

O Allah, make the end of my life the best of my life, and the best of my deeds, their conclusion, and the best of my days, the day on which I shall meet Thee.

O Allah, make death the best of the things we chose not, but which we await; and the grave the best dwelling in which we shall dwell – and, then death, make best that which follows death.

– Ahmad Kamal[19]

The difficult test

Of a surety we will test you with something of fear and hunger, loss of life, or the fruits of your toil.

But give glad tidings to those who patiently persevere.

– *Qur'an*[20]

The Qur'an repeatedly asserts that life is a test. It makes no pretence that the trials and tribulations that life has to offer are significant and, at times, difficult to bear; we are also reminded that in all cases these are surmountable. Undoubtedly one of the most distressing experiences for any individual is the loss of a loved one. However, loss need not be a completely negative experience as it represents an occasion to reflect on social and spiritual relationships, and indeed on the purpose and meaning of life itself. A Sufi master will speak of bereavement as offering the opportunity to reach the station of *Sabr* – an Arabic term that denotes the state of constant and unconditional contentment with the divine decree. *Sabr* represents one of the greatest heights of spiritual development that a Muslim can attain. It is this quality that the bereaved family will be encouraged to practise and develop by fellow community members. Perhaps unsurprisingly, not all practices conform to religious dictates; for example, Islam strongly prohibits wailing following death, yet the practice continues in many quarters. This pre-Islamic custom that originally existed to express the sense of loss felt perhaps continues as a vehicle to inform fellow community members that their support will be needed in the weeks and months ahead.

Loss of offspring, irrespective of their stage of development, is a most trying experience. Here, in addition to encouraging *Sabr*, community members will attempt to comfort the bereaved by reminding them that children are pure and innocent and therefore are assured of paradise.

Radio ga ga

Caller: 'What about a woman who has a miscarriage? Some people say that, well, you shouldn't get too upset, because the loss isn't real – it's not like the death of a child.'

Panellist: 'The pain and loss can be very real; as couples see their hopes fade away. We should be sensitive, recognising the difficulty of the situation. For those who remain resolute, thinking good of Allah, there is the deeply comforting tradition of the Prophet (may Allah bless him and grant him peace):

'By Him in whose hand is my soul, the miscarried foetus draws its mother into Paradise by its umbilical cord, when she seeks her reward [for the loss] from Allah.'

– Radio Ramadan

Dear Uncle

We here, so many miles away, are with you, in this difficult hour. You *must* remember, my dearest uncle, that what has happened is by Allah's decree – a plan that we cannot always understand. As for Sami, he is now free, having escaped the difficulties of this world; it is as if we can see him – laughing, playing, with that cheeky grin – rejoicing in his new home, his *real* home. We must wait patiently for the time when we too will finally join him – that final union. Your pain, our pain, Allah knows is real – but, dear uncle, take solace in the words of our Prophet (may Allah bless him and grant him peace):

When a child of a servant of Allah passes away, Allah says to the angels: 'Did you take away the apple of My servant's eye?' They reply: 'Yes.' He, the Almighty, then asks: 'What did My servant say?' They say: 'He praised you and said: "Unto Allah we belong and unto Allah will we return".' At this Allah says: 'Build for My servant a mansion in Paradise – and call it the House of Praise.'

(Sami died suddenly and unexpectedly, aged six.)

An activist model

The immediate pre- and post-death rituals encourage a 'hands-on' approach to dying and death.[21] Close relatives and friends will typically participate in the physical and spiritual care of the dying, and take a lead role in organising and performing the post-death rites of washing, shrouding and burying the deceased. Ensuring that these rights are performed in a quick, efficient and dignified manner is an important consideration for the family and will occupy much of the initial post-death period. The prescribed rituals during this period provide great stability at a time that has the potential to cause much disorientation; the active involvement in the care of the deceased ensures that the feelings of numbness and denial described by Bowlby in his phase model of bereavement are unusual among Muslims.[22]

Mourning is usually for three days, during which community members will visit the household of the deceased. Two or three hundred visitors during this time is not unusual. The mood is serious and reflective, yet one in which positive aspects of the deceased's personal narrative are freely and frequently expounded.

Formal and informal prayers for the individual's welfare in the life to come are a central theme; visitors will also pray that immediate family members be blessed with achieving the station of *Sabr*. The community support available means that, for those with well established family and community networks, recourse to medical services is infrequently needed. The traditional supportive role of medical staff in such situations may thus be inadvertently challenged, resulting in feelings of unease and alienation on the part of the doctor. Understanding of Muslim death customs should prevent such a response occurring.

Comforting thoughts

'Whenever I stopped reciting [from the Qur'an], she would rouse somewhat, as if to say, "Carry on! Don't stop!" She died peacefully – whilst I recited.'
– Schoolteacher, reflecting on the death of his mother

In the case of widows, the mourning period is approximately 19 weeks, by which time it should be apparent if the widow is carrying her husband's offspring. The period of mourning for a pregnant woman terminates on delivery, irrespective of the duration since her husband's death. In our experience, this mourning period is usually respected, with women remaining primarily within the marital home. Many, however, are unaware of the religious dispensation allowing travel for seeking medical care, resulting in poor attendance for clinic appointments. A proactive, yet flexible, approach to dealing with this issue is to be encouraged. In most cases, it should be possible to offer a more convenient appointment. Where delay is detrimental, education regarding the religious obligation to seek medical attention (perhaps using leaflets written in conjunction with local religious leaders) and greater use of domiciliary services are the key.

Enduring relationships

Within some philosophies, death marks the end. For the adherents of such a philosophy, death will also mark the end of relationships that were once enjoyed. Islam takes a radically different view, for not only do relationships continue, it is considered possible to assist the deceased in their further journeying. This honouring of the deceased is a value that many Muslims nurture from early childhood, such as regularly visiting graveyards where loved ones have been laid to rest. The greeting used on entering the graveyard, *Assalamu Alaikum* meaning 'peace be with you', is the same as that used to greet the living. The prayer that follows emphasises the fact that reunion will take place.

Waiting patiently

On entering a graveyard the Prophet (may Allah bless him and grant him peace) recommended the following words:

'Peace be with you, O you dwellers of these abodes – believers and Muslims. May Allah have mercy on those of you who were first to die and those who were last. We will, whenever Allah wills, join you. I beseech Allah for salvation for you and us.'[23]

If the deceased had any outstanding religious obligations, such as the pilgrimage to Mecca (Hajj), family members will try to fulfil these requirements on their behalf. Also considered important is the need to maintain relationships and friendships that the individual enjoyed when alive. Perpetuating social networks of this kind has also been shown to be important to primary care medical staff. Finally, it is important to be aware that the deceased can be credited with good after leaving this world. Family and friends, by contributing to such metaphysical memorial funds, have the opportunity to make an enduring legacy to a loved one, wherever and whenever they feel the need.

Recurrent Hajj syndrome

Nazir, a middle-aged accountant, made preparations for his fourth Hajj (pilgrimage to Mecca) in as many years. Having completed his own, he had performed the sacred rite on behalf of his late parents, they themselves not having had the means to make the journey during their lifetime. One debt now remained – Hajj on behalf of his grandfather.

Post-mortems and organ transplants

For novel matters that are not explicitly dealt with in Islamic Law, Muslim jurists are required to study the issue in question and using the principles enshrined within the Qur'an and *Hadith* arrive at a legal opinion, known as a *Fatwa*. It is important to appreciate that a *Fatwa* is an opinion and therefore not binding; thus one can expect a broad range of views on a given question (*see* Chapter 4). This is the case with post-mortem examinations and organ transplantation.

The majority opinion is that post-mortem examinations are not allowed. The reasons for this include the fact that the post-mortem will inevitably delay the burial. Second, some Muslims believe that it may be possible for the deceased to still perceive pain. This is based on the statement of the Prophet Muhammad that 'To break the bone of a dead person is like breaking the bone of a living person'.[24] This tradition is, however, more commonly interpreted as referring to the need to continue to respect the dead.

Where the law of the land demands post-mortem examinations; that is, at the coroner's request, Muslims have no choice but to comply. In this case, informing the coroner's officer that the deceased is a Muslim may speed up the process, as many coroners are now aware of Muslim sensitivities. There is, however, the wider issue of whether the UK's coroner's service is in need of reform so that it more accurately reflects the diversity of opinion on post-mortem examinations found in modern-day pluralist societies.[25] Having first-hand experience of the intense pain and suffering that such state intrusions may cause, we would very strongly urge that the criteria for compulsory post-mortem for Muslims, and perhaps also the Orthodox Jewish community, be restricted to those cases in which there is a genuine medico-legal need.[26] For post-mortem examinations that clinicians consider desirable for educational or other purposes, it is important that it is made explicit that family members have a free choice in the matter, and that their views will be respected.

With respect to organ transplants opinion is more divided. For the reasons cited above, many oppose the donating of organs. Further it is argued that since life is a 'trust', one has no right to 'donate' any part of one's body to someone else. This view is particularly common among Muslims of South Asian origin. An increasing number of Muslims, however, are of the view that in cases where organ donation may save life then it is allowed, even desirable, on the basis of the Islamic doctrine that 'necessity allows the prohibited'. An important *Fatwa* from the UK-based Muslim Law (*Shariah*) Council in 1995 was strongly supportive of Muslims donating organs, and is gradually contributing to changing perceptions in relation to the legitimacy of donating organs.[27]

On a practical level, we suggest that discussions concerning organ transplantation are initiated by the transplant team, included in which should be personnel familiar with Muslim anxieties, allowing these concerns to be addressed accurately and sensitively. Such liaison workers may also have a key role to play in the aftermath of organ donation or transplant, exploring and allaying any feelings of guilt that may ensue.

Summary

- Muslim death and bereavement customs are strongly shaped by religious teachings; an understanding of this narrative is important to allow care to be appropriately delivered.
- Family members are strongly encouraged to participate in the care of the dying; where possible Muslims should be allowed and encouraged to take a 'hands-on' approach to the care of dying friends and relatives.
- Relaxation of hospital visiting regulations would facilitate this.
- A quick burial is encouraged. Barriers to this include delay in having death certificates issued and registering the death, the need for post-mortem examinations, and difficulties in burying the deceased at weekends and on public holidays.
- Difficulties in observing death rites are likely to have detrimental effects on the bereavement process that ensues; Muslim bereavement remains an under-researched area.
- On organ transplantation, the Muslim community expresses mixed views. Any campaign aimed at encouraging organ donation by Muslims should reflect an appreciation of Islamic teaching on the subject.

Acknowledgements

Some of the material in this chapter has been reproduced, with permission, from a paper published in the *Journal of the Royal Society of Medicine* [Sheikh A (1998) Death and dying – a Muslim perspective. *J R Soc Med.* **91**: 138–40].

References

1 Ali YA (1938) *The Meaning of the Glorious Quran*; **2**: 185 (trans modified). Dar al-Kitab: Cairo.

2 al-Ghazali AH (1995) *The Remembrance of Death and the Afterlife.* Islamic Texts Society: Cambridge.

3 Sheikh A (1998) Death and dying – a Muslim perspective. *J R Soc Med*; **91**: 138–40.

4 an-Nawawi (1976) *Forty Hadith*, p. 26. The Holy Koran Publishing House: Damascus.

5 Gatrad AR (1994) Muslim customs surrounding death, bereavement, postmortem examinations, and organ transplants. *BMJ.* **309**: 521–3.

6 Ali YA (1938) *The Meaning of the Glorious Quran*; **36**: 51–8 (trans modified). Dar al-Kitab: Cairo.

7 Gatrad AR, Sheikh A (2002) Palliative care for Muslims and issues before death. *Int J Palliat Nurs*; **8**: 526–31.

8 Gatrad AR, Sadiq R, Sheikh A (2003) Multifaith chaplaincy. *Lancet*; **362**: 748.

9 Gatrad AR, Browne E, Sheikh A (2004) Developing multi-faith chaplaincy. *Arch Dis Child*; **89**: 504–5.

10 Lie ASJ (2006) Multi-faith chaplaincy. In: Gatrad R, Brown E, Sheikh A (eds). *Palliative Care for South Asians: Muslims Hindus and Sikhs*, pp. 155–66. Quay: London.

11 Sheikh A (1997) Quiet room is needed in hospitals for prayer and reflection. *BMJ*; **315**: 1625.

12 Sheikh A, Gatrad AR, Sheikh U, Panesar SS, Shafi S. (2004) Hospital chaplaincy units show bias towards Christianity. *BMJ*; **329**: 626.

13 Gatrad AR, Sheikh A (2002) Palliative care for Muslims and issues after death. *Int J Palliat Nurs*; **8**: 594–7.

14 Nielsen JS (1988) Muslims in Britain and local authority responses. In: T Gerholm, YG Lithman (eds) *The New Islamic Presence in Western Europe.* Mansell: London.

15 Firth S (2006) South Asian perspectives on bereavement. In: Gatrad R, Brown E, Sheikh A (eds). *Palliative Care for South Asians: Muslims Hindus and Sikhs*, pp. 167–82. Quay: London.

16 Charlton R, Dolman E (1995) Bereavement: a protocol for primary care. *Br J Gen Pract*; **45**: 427–30.

17 Woof WR, Carter YH (1997) The grieving adult and the general practitioner: a literature review in two parts (part 1). *Br J Gen Pract*; **47**: 443–8.

18 Woof WR, Carter YH (1997) The grieving adult and the general practitioner: a literature review in two parts (part 2). *Br J Gen Pract*; **47**: 509–14.

19 Kamal A (1964) *The Sacred Journey*, p. 32. Allen and Unwin: London.

20 Ali YA (1938) *The Meaning of the Glorious Quran*; **2**: 155–7 (trans modified). Dar al-Kitab: Cairo.

21 Gatrad AR, Brown E, Notta H, Sheikh A (2003). Palliative care needs of minorities. *BMJ*; **327**:176–7.

22 Bowlby J (1983) *Loss: sadness and depression. Attachment and Loss*, vol 3. Basic Books: New York.

23 Cited in: Badawi J (1993) *Selected Prayers*, pp. 60–1. Ta Ha: London.

24 al-Asqalani AIH (1996) *Bulugh al-Maram*, pp. 199–200. Dar-us-Salam Publications: Riyadh.

25 Sheikh A, Gatrad AR, Dhami S (1999) Culturally sensitive care for the dying is a basic human right. *BMJ*; **319**: 1073.

26 Pounder D (1999) The coroner service. *BMJ*; **318**: 1502–3.

27 Anon (1996) The Muslim Law (Shariah) Council and organ transplants. *Accid Emerg Nurs*; **4**: 73–5.

CHAPTER 10

Conclusions: breaking barriers, building bridges

(★ *Aziz Sheikh and Abdul Rashid Gatrad*

Religion and health share a rich and intricate past; their present interrelationship is arguably all the more intriguing. For not only do they meet at the great turning points of life, the junctures of birth and death, but religion continues to profoundly influence and shape notions of health and disease for very many people. '*Omnis natura Deo loquitur*' (the whole of nature speaks of God)[1] is the framework within which the man of faith sees the universe around him; matters to do with health must of necessity then fall within the scope of this world-view. In this work, we have sought to build on the growing corpus of academic and lay writing on the interface between faith and health by focusing attention on the traditions, experiences, hopes and concerns of Muslims – Western Europe and North America's fastest growing religion. An appreciation of Islam, and its central narrative, then is vital to understanding these peoples and the ways in which they experience and comprehend this sacred interface.

But understanding Islam, for the Western educated health professional at least, is difficult. When seeking to relate to his or her Muslim patient important barriers stand in the way. First, there is the problem of institutional racism embedded firmly within European and American culture.[2] The former British Home Secretary, The Right Honourable Jack Straw MP, for example, acknowledged that the National Health Service is 'a long-established, white-dominated organisation [which] is liable to have procedures, practices and a culture that tend to exclude or to disadvantage non-White people'.[3] The net effect is that healthcare professionals will typically have ingrained within them, often subconsciously, the belief that the lifestyles and mannerisms of coloured peoples are inferior to those of the White majority.[4,5]

There is in addition the difficulty of how, and to what degree, those educated in a secular biomedical model of healthcare, which takes as its starting point Parkin's 'spiritless cadaver',[6] can relate to and understand those who bring with them very different notions of existence. As post-Renaissance man lost his integrated vision of existence, he chose to concentrate his energies and enquiries on the physical and material. Reduced to an accident of history, he turned outwards in search of fulfilment. Natural then that science, now synonymous with domination, mastery and exploitation of the earth and her resources, should rise to a position of supreme importance.[7,8] Medicine retained an important position within the mechanistic universe rapidly being constructed,[9-11] its role now though very different, for no longer was it engaged in delivering the 'holism' of the Semitic faiths or the 'balance' of the Taoist. Rather, it had now become pitted in battle – the battle for survival. Any remnants of belief about matters transcendent became, and remain, coloured with the immutable dichotomy of 'sacred' and 'mundane'.

Being faced with Muslims who have never recognised such divisions is therefore challenging and complex. For theirs is a vision that acknowledges the tri-partite nature of man, comprising *spiritus*, *anima* and *corpus*, and one in which unity reigns supreme. This unity they see extending beyond their immediacy, finding resonance in the world around them. Charged with fulfilling the time-honoured role of trustee and custodian, all is, and must be, 'sacred'.

And then there is the widespread, pernicious and persistent problem of Islamophobia.[12-14] A millennium of hostilities directed against Muslims and their religion has not been without consequence.[15,16] Dismissed initially as a 'heretical faith', the Western powers maintained that Muhammad was 'cruel and crafty, lustful and ignorant', motivating his followers through the 'crude outpourings of the Koran'. The Oriental attack took on a more subtle tone during the imperialist era, arguing that although Muhammad was 'undoubtedly sincere' it must nonetheless be concluded that it was his religion that was responsible for the 'backwardness' of Muslims *vis-à-vis* their colonial rulers.[17] The attacks continue almost unabated, the tried and trusted headline of an 'Islamic bomb', or yet another 'Muslim fundamentalist on the killing rampage' are enticement enough it seems for those obsessed with feeding past prejudices. Little wonder then that almost endemic within Western society are the beliefs that Islam denigrates women, is anti-progressive, and a religion of terror and extremism. The global 'threat from Islam' is thus to many a Western mind both real and imminent;[18] these have been added credence by the recent wave of terrorist attacks inflicted by those who pervert the true teachings of the faith.[19,20]

The all-too-familiar stories of misunderstanding, prejudice and discrimination that we have heard testify to the difficulties that lie in the path of those wishing to deliver culturally competent and sensitive care. Take, for example, the Turkish bookseller who, after his wife had been delivered of their third and 'final' child by Caesarean section, asked if Islam was really so despised by 'the West' that the surgeon's knife had too been recruited in the battle to curb Muslim numbers. Or the elderly Afghani, on being made aware of the animal gelatine component of the antibiotic capsules he had been prescribed, asked how his general practitioner could have made such an important mistake. Or the middle-aged Kenyan car mechanic who, wiping a tear from his eye, enquired why the medical profession had subjected his elderly mother to the pains of a post-mortem – was the caring profession really so insensitive?

But despite the sorry picture painted, and the barriers identified, our prognosis is not necessarily bleak. For those who see a need to bridge gulfs, there must always exist certain rays of hope. Take, for example, the burgeoning medical interest in issues to do with race, ethnicity and culture, both conceptual and applied, which has led to considerable progress in understanding the impact of such factors on issues to do with health and healthcare delivery.[21–26] It must, however, be admitted that this work is yet still in its infancy, and its role in shaping medical education, research, clinical care and health policy remains marginal.

There is too a growing belief that despite all its breathtaking successes the reductionism that characterises biomedicine impoverishes our conception of human beings. Through focusing on only the temporal side of man, and in seeking to conquer rather than concur with nature, it is suggested that modern medicine has severed its links with the health beliefs of a diverse array of cultures and almost all health belief models constructed hitherto.[27] For whether we choose to study Indian Vedic medicine,[28] ancient Chinese medicine,[29,30] or indeed the medicine of Antiquity,[31] from which biomedicine claims its origins, notions of spirituality and the metaphysical dimension of existence have figured strongly. The once lone voice of Nasr,[32,33] the brilliant exponent of traditionalism, asserting that medicine needs to 'rediscover the anatomy of being', is it seems gaining momentum and wider acceptance.

In the United States in particular, it now appears that a *vox populi* has begun to make itself heard arguing for more explicit connections between religion and health to be re-established.[34,35] Research suggests that public belief in the benefits to health of religious faith and practices are high.[36,37] Also noteworthy is that there is some evidence to suggest that a smaller, though significant, proportion of the medical community may also subscribe to this view. For example, of 296 physicians surveyed during the 1996 American Academy of Family Physicians meeting, 99% were of the opinion that religious beliefs can have healing effects, and over 70% were of the opinion that the prayers of others could help a patient's recovery.[34] The subsequent religion-health outcome debate that is currently afoot in America sends ripples of uncertainties through those who had, so they thought, buried religion once and for all.

Outcome measures considered have thus included indices of psychological well-being, where much of the work to date has been concentrated,[37,38] and lifestyle factors important to health such as cigarette consumption,[39] alcohol consumption[40] and marital status.[41] Not surprisingly perhaps, religious involvement has been shown to have a health protective role, being associated with a lower risk of mental health problems and a lifestyle favourable to promoting health. More recently, interest has begun to focus on the effects of religious practice on physical health. Here, once again, evidence points in favour of religious practices being associated with a diverse array of health benefits, such as better obstetric outcome,[42] lower blood pressure,[43] reduced risk of cancer[44] and increased overall life expectancy.[45–47]

Some of these health benefits may in part be explained by factors such as differing demographics, health habits and social support among the religiously active. Nonetheless, the benefits to health are shown on balance to persist in studies that have attempted to control for such potential confounding factors. Further, early work exploring the impact of religion on health service utilisation also seems to suggest a close relationship between the two, with lower consulting rates, lower hospital admission rates and decreased length of hospital stay among those who express a religious commitment.[49,50]

We also take comfort from recent positive soundings from the Council of Europe, re-emphasising that patients have a right to have their religious beliefs respected. Such positive sentiments are also central to *The Patient's Charter*,[51] finding echoes in the principles embedded within the General Medical Council guidelines *Duties of a Doctor*[52] and *Good Medical Practice*.[53] The greater willingness of research charities and biomedical journals to fund and report research to do with matters religious, and the willingness from the Department of Health to support and work with faith groups,[54] suggest to us that religion is set to assume a more culturally civic position among the medical profession. While the proposition that the 'wall of separation' between religion and medicine may soon be demolished seems somewhat premature,[55] it is clear that the longstanding dialogue between religion and health still has much to offer.[56–60]

As Europe come to terms with its past, there is a greater willingness from the British establishment to promote dialogue and discussion with Muslims about relationships between Muslims and the West. Fundamental differences in outlook may of course exist, but this should not prevent either community from recognising the very many points of similarities – the common Judeo-Christian origin of our societies, our respect for learning and the institutions of the family to mention but a few examples. The positive calls for dialogue from the likes of HRH The Prince of Wales[61,62] and the former British Prime Minister[63] have also provided cause for optimism. Most reassuring of all, however, are those small gestures – the kind midwife who after delivering the young Indian accountant of her firstborn asks, 'Can I cover you?', the offer of state circumcision displayed on the paediatric ward notice board, the water jug in the surgery lavatory, those touching electronic *Eid* cards from colleagues and a Secretary of State for Health greeting his Muslim audience with '*Assalamu-Alaikum*'.[64] Small gestures, but ones that we feel bode well for the future.

This work has attempted to explore and, in the process, unveil a certain face of the Muslim patient hitherto hidden from the view of many. We have, with the help of our co-authors, tried to provide healthcare professionals with the key that allows access to the essence, or *qalb*, of the Muslim's being. And if we have succeeded, to whatever extent, we have, we believe, contributed to the breaking of the most important of barriers and the building of the most crucial of bridges.

What comes from the lips reaches the ears.
What comes from the heart reaches the heart.

– Arab proverb [65]

References

1 Hugo of St Victor *Eruditio didascalia.* Cited in: Nasr SH (1997) *Man and Nature: the spiritual crisis in modern man,* p. 10. ABC: Chicago.
2 Macpherson W (1999) *Report for the Stephen Lawrence Inquiry.* The Stationery Office: London.
3 Straw J (1999) *House of Commons Hansard Debates,* 24 February, col 391. HMSO: London.
4 Ahmad WIU (1993) *'Race' and Health in Contemporary Britain.* OUP: Buckingham.
5 Coker N (ed) (2001) *Racism in Medicine: an agenda for change.* King's Fund: London.
6 Parkin D (1999) Suffer many healers. In: JR Hinnells, R Porter (eds) *Religion, Health and Suffering,* p. 434. Kegan Paul: London.
7 Bacon F (1995) In: T Anderson (ed) *The New Organon.* Bobbs Merrill: Indianapolis.
8 Russell BA (1979) *A History of Western Philosophy.* Allen and Unwin: London.
9 Butt N (1991) *Science and Muslim Societies.* Grey Seal: London.
10 Porter R (1970) *The Greatest Benefit to Mankind,* pp. 270–396. Harper Collins, London.
11 Foucault M (1973) *The Birth of the Clinic.* Tavistock: London.
12 Runnymede Trust (1997) *Islamophobia: a challenge for us all.* Runnymede Trust: London.
13 Weller P, Fieldman A, Purdam K (2001). *Religious Discrimination in England and Wales,* p. 220. Home Office Research Development and Statistics Directorate: London.
14 Richardson R (ed). (2004) *Islamophobia: Issues, Challenges and Actions: a report by the commission on British Muslims and Islamophobia.* Trentham Books: Stoke-on-Trent.
15 Gunny A (1996) *Images of Islam: eighteenth century writings.* Grey Seal: London.
16 Thomson A (1989) *Blood on the Cross.* Ta Ha: London.
17 Eaton G (1985) *Islam and the Destiny of Man,* pp. 9–30. George Allen and Unwin: London.
18 Esposito JL (1992) *The Islamic Threat.* OUP: Oxford.
19 Halliday F (2001) *Two Hours that Shook the World: September 11, 2001, causes and consequences.* Saqi: London.
20 Sheikh A (2001) *Understanding Islam.* Reform Magazine. Available from: http://www.urc.org.uk/reform_magazine/articles/understanding_islam/index.htm
21 Qureshi B (1989) *Transcultural Medicine.* Kluwer: London.
22 Leff J (1988) *Psychiatry Around the Globe: a transcultural view.* Gaskell Press, Penguin: London.
23 Littlewood R, Lipsedge M (1982) *Aliens and Alienists: ethnic minorities and psychiatry.* Penguin: London.
24 Helman CG (2001) *Culture, Health and Illness.* Arnold: London.

25 Arora S, Coker N, Gillam S, Ismail H (2000) *Improving the Health of Black and Minority Ethnic Groups: a guide for PCGs.* King's Fund: London.

26 Bhopal RS (2007) *Ethnicity, Race, and Health in Multicultural Societies: foundations for better epidemiology, public health, and health care.* OUP: Oxford.

27 Sheikh A (1999) Religion, health and suffering. *J R Soc Med*; **92**: 600–1.

28 Zyst KG (1993) *Religious Medicine: the history and evolution of Indian medicine.* Transaction Publishers: New Brunswick.

29 Unschuld P (1985) *Medicine in China: a history of ideas.* University of California Press: Berkeley.

30 Bray F (1997) Chinese health beliefs. In: JR Hinnells, R Porter (eds) *Religion, Health and Suffering*, pp. 187–211. Kegan Paul: London.

31 Singer C, Underwood EA (1962) *A Short History of Medicine.* Clarendon Press: Oxford.

32 Nasr SH (1997) *Man and Nature: the spiritual crisis in modern man.* ABC: Chicago.

33 Nasr SH (1997) *The Need for a Sacred Science.* Curzon Press: Richmond.

34 Sloan RP, Bagiella P, Powell T (1999) Religion, spirituality and medicine. *Lancet*; **353**: 664–7.

35 King DE, Bushwick B (1994) Beliefs and attitudes of hospital inpatients about faith healing and prayer. *J Fam Pract*; **39**: 349–52.

36 Koenig HG (1999) Religion and medicine. *Lancet*; **353**: 1803.

37 Koenig HG, McCullough ME, Larson DB (2001) *Handbook of Religion and Health.* OUP: Oxford.

38 Koenig HG, Cohen HJ (2002) *The Link between Religion and Health: psychoneuroimmunology and the faith factor.* OUP: Oxford.

39 Koenig HG, George LK, Cohen HJ, Hays JC, Larson DB, Blazer DG (1998) The relationship between religious activities and cigarette smoking in older adults. *J Gerontol A Biol Sci Med Sci*; **53**: M426–34.

40 Koenig HG, George LK, Meador KG, Blazer DG, Ford SM (1994) Religious practices and alcoholism in a southern adult population. *Hosp Commun Psychiat*; **45**: 225–31.

41 Strawbridge WJ, Cohen RD, Shema SJ, Kaplan GA (1997) Frequent attendance at religious services and mortality over 28 years. *Am J Public Hlth*; **87**: 957–61.

42 King DE, Hueston W, Rudy M (1994) Religious affiliation and obstetric outcome. *South Med J*; **87**: 1125–8.

43 Koenig HG, George LK, Hays JC, Larson DB, Cohen HJ, Blazer DG (1998) The relationship between religious activities and blood pressure in older adults. *Int J Psychiatry Med*; **28**: 189–213.

44 Rabin BS (1999) Religion and medicine. *Lancet*; **353**: 1803.

45 Hummer RA, Rogers RG, Nam CB, Elison CG (1999) Religious involvement and US adult mortality. *Demography*; **36**: 273–85.

46 Koenig HG, Hays JC, Larson DB, *et al.* (1999) A six year follow-up study of 3968 older adults. *J Gerontol A Biol Sci Med Sci*; **54**: M370–6.

47 Oman D, Reed D (1998) Religion and mortality among the community dwelling elderly. *Am J Public Hlth*; **88**: 1469–75.

48 Kark JD, Shemi G, Friedlander Y, Martin O, Manor O, Blondheim SH (1996) Does religious observance promote health? Secular vs kibbutzim in Israel. *Am J Public Hlth*; **86**: 341–6.

49 Koenig HG, Larson DB (1998) Use of hospital services, religious attendance, and religious affiliation. *South Med J*; **91**: 925–32.

50 Sicher F, Targ E, Moore D, Smith HJ (1998) A randomised double-blind study of the effects of distant healing in a population with advanced AIDS: report of a small-scale study. *West J Med*; **169**: 356–63.

51 Department of Health (1999) *The Patient's Charter*. DoH: London.

52 General Medical Council (1995) *Duties of a Doctor*. GMC: London.

53 General Medical Council (2006) *Good Medical Practice*. GMC: London.

54 Anon (1998) Faith, health and communities. *Our Healthier Nation Target*; **31**: 2–4.

55 Matthews DA, Larson DB (1997) Faith and medicine: reconciling the twin traditions of healing. *Mind/body Med*; **2**: 3–6.

56 Henley A, J Schott (1999) (eds) *Culture, Religion and Patient Care in a Multi-ethnic Society*. Age Concern England: London.

57 Firth S (1997) *Dying, Death and Bereavement in a British Hindu Community*. Peeters: Leuven.

58 Spitzer J (2003) *Caring for Jewish Patients*. Radcliffe: Oxon.

59 Mynors G, Ghalamkari H, Beaumont S, Powell S, McGee P (eds) (2004) *Informed Choice in Medicine Taking: drugs of porcine origin and clinical alternatives*. Medicines Partnership: London.

60 Gatrad R, Brown E, Sheikh A (eds) (2006) *Palliative Care for South Asians: Muslims, Hindus and Sikhs*. Quay: London.

61 HRH The Prince of Wales (1993) *Islam and the West*. Speech delivered in Oxford, 27 October.

62 HRH The Prince of Wales (2006) *Unity in Faith*. Speech delivered in Cairo, 21 March.

63 The Right Honourable Tony Blair MP (1999) *Fighting for a Society of Shared Values and Human Dignity*. Speech delivered in London, 5 May.

64 The Right Honourable Frank Dobson MP (1998) Speaking at the Muslim Doctors and Dentists Association and The Islamic Medical Association of North America Annual Conference in Birmingham, 27 June.

65 Cited in: Ahmed AS (1993). *Living Islam*, p. 211. BBC Books: London.

Appendices and Glossary

Islam and medicine on the World Wide Web

☪ *Saddaf Alam*

This guide aims to give quick and easy access to high quality material of potential relevance to the care of Muslim patients from the web. The first section contains general information and some useful medical search engines and compendiums. The following sections concentrate more on aspects of relevance in dealing with Muslim patients as well as resources on aspects of Islam and health.

In general, most of these sites are well established, with URLs that have been unchanged for sometime. Where possible, sites have been evaluated according to their design, aesthetics, content, accessibility and quality of site maintenance.

Section 1: General Medical

He@lth information on the Internet
www.hioti.org
A Royal Society of Medicine and Wellcome Trust collaboration. Provides an online resource, newsletter and discussion on the best health related web-sites.

HealthFinder
www.healthfinder.gov
US government site containing details of 'reliable' health information on the net.

Emory Health
www.medweb.emory.edu/medweb

A catalogue of health related web-sites maintained by the Emory Health Services library and intended to provide information for education, research and as a patient resource.

National Library of Medicine
www.nlm.nih.gov
For those interested in searching the biomedical literature. It allows free access to Medline, Cancernet and many other important medical databases.

OMNI
www.omni.ac.uk
UK gateway to filtered medical and health related web-sites.

World Health Organization
www.who.ch
An easy to use site that provides reliable information on issues relating to global healthcare.

Section 2: Islam and Muslims

Discover Islam
www.discoverislam.com
A picture is worth a thousand words, as demonstrated by this gallery of 25 posters integrating traditional Islamic art and the latest computer graphics to give an online exhibition on Islam. (These posters can also be ordered online.)

Images of Islam
www.ummah.org.uk/sanders
Some of the photographer Peter Sanders' beautiful images, captured during a lifetime of travel through the Muslim heartland.

Islam City
www.islam.org
All you wanted to know about Islam but were too afraid to ask! Provides an overview of Islam, broadcasts the prayers from Mecca, and much more! The site of choice for the BBC, CNN and ABC.

Islamic Finder
www.islamicfinder.org
Another good database to find your local mosques, and Muslim charities and businesses. Also provides prayer times for countries around the world.

Islamic Interlink
www.islamicinterlink.com

A compendium of Muslim sites and organisations. Also contains information on the Qur'an, Islamic history and the history of the Prophet Muhammad.

Section 3: Islam and Medicine

Contemporary Topics in Islamic Medicine
www.islam-usa.com/iml.html
Dr Shahid Attar's book online; he is the chairman of the Islamic Society of North America's medical ethics committee.

General articles
www.crescentlife.com/contents
Various articles on Islam and health, wellness, mental health, nutrition etc.

Islamic Medicine
www.islamicmedicine.com
Well stocked web-site with articles on a wide variety of health related topics from an Islamic perspective.

Islamic Organisation for Medical Sciences (IOMS)
www.Islamset.com/introd.html
Large and diverse number of articles on various branches of medicine, including mental health, preventative medicine, sexual health etc. The IOMS have also hosted a number of highly respected international seminars on various medical ethical questions, summaries of which appear on this site.

Muslim Philosophy
www.muslimphilosophy.com
Access to a range of articles on philosophy and psychology.

Section 4: Muslim Health Resources

Chaplaincy training
www.islamic-foundation.org.uk
Its education and training unit provide cultural awareness training as well as running courses to help train hospital chaplains.

Cultural Competency
www.med.umich.edu/multicultural/ccp/mpcc
An initiative by the University if Michigan, looking at cultural competency programmes and caring for patients of different nationalities and faiths.

Cyber Hajj
www.islam.org/cybertv/ch18.htm

A feast of multimedia downloads from ABC and CNN that takes you on a virtual pilgrimage to Mecca.

Cyber Muslim Counselling
www.islamonline.net/Question Application/English/Browse.asp
Ask advice from a pool of Muslim social workers and counsellors.

Death and Dying
www.quran.com/fiqhussunnah/4.asp
www.isgka.org/fiqh_death.htm
Information on aspects of dealing with Muslim deaths and burials.

Domestic Violence
www.islamic-knowledge.com/Rights_duties.htm
Articles on abuse, domestic violence, families and rights. Also lists some organisations working in these fields.

Fatwas
www.islamonline.net/fatwaapplication/english/browse.asp
Ever wondered where to turn to ask a question on a particularly thorny issue regarding a Muslim patient? Ask questions to a panel of Muslim scholars (or browse the database of previous questions and answers)

IPCI
www.ipci-iv.co.uk
This charity allows hospitals to order copies of the Holy Qur'an free of charge.

Islamic Culture and Medical Arts
www.nlm.nih.gov/exhibition/islamic_medicine/islamic_oohtml
Emile Savage Smith of the University of Oxford gives an intriguing account of the intricate relationship between medicine and culture in the Islamic world-view. Read her online book, courtesy of the National Library of Medicine.

Islamic Medical Association of South Africa
www.ima.org.za
Produces a number of leaflets and booklets on various aspects of Muslim health considerations, all of which can be ordered online.

Prayer
www.wings.buffalo.edu/sa/muslim/library/salah
An online well illustrated book on performing prayer and ablutions.

APPENDIX 2

Muslim organisations

(★ *Saddaf Alam*

United Kingdom

An-Nisa Society
85 Wembley Hill Road, Wembley,
Middlesex. HA9 8BU.
Tel: 0208 902 0100
(Women's organisation that has also pioneered several successful projects covering
themes such as sex education, sexual abuse and adoption and fostering.)

Association of Muslims with Disabilities,
1 Hawthorn Road, London. NW10 2NE
Tel/Fax: 0208 830 3821

Association of Muslim Lawyers
PO Box 148. High Wycombe. HP13 5WJ
Tel/Fax: 01494 526955

Association of Muslim Schools
1 Evington Lane, Leicester. LE5 5PQ.
Tel: 0116 273 8666
Fax: 0116 273 8777

Federation of Student Islamic Societies (FOSIS)
3 Mapesbury Road, London. NW2 4JD
Tel: 0208 452 4493
Fax: 0208 208 4161
Email: info@fosis.org.uk

Islamic Foundation
Markfield Dawah Centre,
Ratby Lane, Markfield, Leicester. LE67 9RN.
Tel: 01530 244944
Fax: 01530 244946

Islamic Society of Britain (ISB)
PO Box 7539, Birmingham. B10 9AU.
Phone: 0845 087 8766
Email: info@isb.org.uk

Mediconcern
17 Derby Road, Fallowfield, Manchester. M14 6UX
Tel: 0161 292 5788
Fax: 0161 284 2923
Email: info@mediconcern.org.uk

Muslim Child Helpline
0800 071 1786

Muslim Council of Britain (MCB)
PO Box 57 330, London. E1 2WJ
Tel: 0845 262 6786
Fax: 0207 247 7079
Email: admin@mcb.org.uk

Muslim Directory
65A Grosvenor Road, London. W7 1HR
Tel: 0208840 0020
Fax: 0208 840 8819
Email: info@muslimdirectory.co.uk

Muslim Doctors and Dentist Association
2A Bowyer Road, Saltley, Birmingham. B8 1ET.
Tel/Fax: 0121 326 980
Email: gs.mdda@lineonline.net

Muslim Education Trust
130 Stroud Green Road, London. N4 3RZ.
Tel: 0207 272 8502

Muslim Institute
6 Endsleigh Road, London. WC1H 0DS
Tel: 0207 388 2581

Muslim Marriage Guidance Council
The Brighton Islamic Mission,
8 Caburn Road, Hove, Sussex. BN3 6ET.
Tel: 01273 722 438
Fax: 01273 279 439

Muslim Women's Helpline
11 Main Drive, GEC East Lane Estate, Wembley,
Middlesex. HA9 7PX.
Tel: 0208 904 8193

United States

American Muslim Council (AMC)
2nd St NE, Washington DC
Phone: 202 543 0075
Fax: 202 543 0095
Email: amc@amconline.org

Council on American Islamic Relations (CAIR)
New Jersey Ave SE,
Washington, DC 20003-4034
Tel: 202 488 8787
Fax: 202 488 0833
Email: webmaster@cair-net.org

Islamic Circle of North America (ICNA)
166-26, 89th Avenue, Jamaica, NY 11432
Tel: 718 658 1199
Fax: 718 658 1255
Email: info@icna.org

Islamic Medical Association of North America (IMANA)
4121 South Fairview Avenue, Suite 203
Downers Grove, IL 60515
Tel: 708 852 2122
Fax: 708 852 2151
Email: IMANA@aol.com

Islamic Society of North America (ISNA)
6555 South 750 East, PO Box 38,
Plainsfield, IN 46168
Phone: 317 839 8157
Fax: 317 839 1840
Email: syeeds@isna.net

Muslim Public Affairs Committee (MPAC)
3010 Wilshire Boulevard, #217, Los Angeles,
California 90010
Tel: 213 383 3443
Email: salam@mpac.org

Muslim Student Association of US and Canada
PO Box 18612, Washington, DC 20036
Phone: 703 820 7900
Fax: 703 820 7888
Email: info@msa-natl.org

Canada

Canadian Islamic Congress
420 Erb Street West, Suite 424,
Waterloo, Ontario. N2L 6K6.
Tel: 519 746 1242
Fax: 519 746 2929

Islamic Families Social Services Association
Unit #85, 4003-98 Street, Edmonton. AB T6E 6M8
Tel/Fax: 780 430 9220
Email: info@ifsaa.ca

Islamic Information Foundation
8 Laurel Avenue, Halifax, NS, B3M 2P6
Phone: 902 445 2494
Fax: 902 445 2494

Islamic Social Services Association
4202 Roblin Blvd, Winnipeg,
Manitoba, R3R 0E7.
Tel: 1-866-239-ISSA (toll free)
Fax: 204 896 1694

Europe

Association of Muslim Communities in the Netherlands
Daguerrestraat 2, 2561 TT Den Haag
Tel/Fax: 00-31-70-427656

Federation of Islamic Organisations in Europe
PO Box MAR005, Markfield, LE67 9RY

Tel: 01530 245913
Fax: 01530 245919

Federation of Islamic Organisations in France
20, Rue de Prevote, 93120 La Courneuve.
Tel: 00-33-1-43111060
Fax: 00-33-1-43111061
Email: uoif@club-interet.fr

Federation of Social Organisations in Ukraine
P.O. Box 599/8
Kiev 126, Ukraine
Tel: 380-44-4434485
Fax: 380-44-4496546
Email: arraid@carrier.kiev.ua

Islamic Cultural Centre
Toyenbekken 24, Oslo 0188
Tel: 22-172591
Fax: 22-176580
Email: info@Islamic.no

Islamic Society of Finland
PL/Box 87, 00101 Helsinki
Tel/Fax: 00-359-9-2782551/3
Email: chehav@dlc.fi

Islamiska Forbundet I Sverige
Ringvagen 135 NB, 116 61 Stockholm
Tel: 00-46-8-6402468
Fax: 00-46-8-6410465
Email: ogg869u@tninet.se

Muslim Association of Denmark
Blommevangen 12,2. Tv
2765 Smorum
Tel: 00-45-44-650079
Fax: 00-45-44-650274
Email: alfarra@mail.tele.dk

Muslim League Switzerland
Ligue des Musulmans de Suisse (L.M.S)
Case Postale 1861, CH 2002 Neuchatel.
Tel/Fax: 00-41-329-314595
Email: rabita@rabita.ch

Organisation for Education and Culture in Germany
Islamisches Buildings Werk (I.B.W.)
Roon Street 39-41, 50674 Koln
Tel: 00-49-(0) 22-1-2761680
Fax: 00-49-(0) 22-1-2761681
Email: info@ibw-deutschland.de

The Cultural Council
Wurlitzergrasse 51/11
1160 Wien, Austria
Tel: 43-14848995
Fax: 43-14812376
Email: lk@Vienna.at

The Muslim Association for Cultural Exchange in Belgium
B.P. 389, Bruxelles 1010
Tel/Fax: 00-32-43-427754
Email: lidben.benn@worldonline.de

Unione Delle Communita Ed Organizzazioni Islamiche in Italia
Via Padova 38, 20127, Milano
Tel: 39-01-83660253
Fax: 39-01-83661707
Email: ucoii@uno.it

Union of Muslim Students in Czech Republic
PO Box 29, Posta Praha 618
16300 Praha 6
Tel: 00-420-2-49681
Fax: 00-420-2-3022842
Email: ashraf@fsv.cvut.cz

Glossary

abtest: Turkish term for the ritual ablution that precedes the five daily prayers (*see wudu*).

Adhan: the call to prayer. Within this call are incorporated the basic tenets of Islam – the belief that Allah alone is worthy of worship and that Muhammad is the Messenger of Allah. The call concludes with the reminder that true felicity is dependent on the realisation of this basic truth. It is customary to whisper the words of the Adhan into the right ear of the newborn immediately after birth.

afiya: a state of wholeness and total well-being.

Allah: the Supreme Being. The term Allah is unique in that it does not have any gender connotation and does not allow a plural form.

Aqiqah: the celebratory sacrifice of an animal on the birth of a child. The meat is distributed between family members, friends and the poor.

Assalamu-Alaikum: peace be with you. The greeting used among Muslims when greeting their living or their dead. It is customary to reciprocate this prayer.

bimaristan: used to describe both fixed and mobile hospitals. (*maristan*: hospital for the insane).

dar'-al-mafsadah: a term from the Islamic legal system which refers to the ethical principle of the warding off of harm.

darurat: necessities or essential actions which are required to preserve the six universal values: religion, life, sanity, property, lineage and human dignity. These are, by definition, essential to normal order in society as well as to the survival and spiritual well-being of individuals, so much so that their destruction and collapse will precipitate chaos and collapse of normal order in society.

dhikr: the remembrance of Allah.

Eid: the major days of celebration of the Islamic calendar. *Eid-ul-Fitr* is the festival that follows the Ramadan fast, falling on the 1st of Shawwal. *Eid-ul-Adha* is the festival of sacrifice that coincides with the last day of the Hajj. This occurs on the 10th of Dhul Hijjah.

fard: an obligatory religious duty.

Fatwa: a formal religious edict.

Fitra: the innate state of purity and goodness with which humans enter this world.

ghusl: purificatory wash that needs to be taken after ejaculation, sexual intercourse, the end of menstruation and death.

Hadith: the sayings of the Prophet Muhammad.

hajiyyat: that which is needed to help maintain the six universals without hardship. Complementary interests are not an independent category as they also seek to protect and promote the essential interests, albeit in a secondary capacity. These are defined as benefits, which seek to remove severity and hardship that do not pose a threat to the very survival of normal order.

Hajj (Hadj): the annual pilgrimage to The Sacred Mosque in Mecca is required of all adult Muslims at least once in a lifetime. There is an exemption for those with poor health or inadequate finances. Is also used as an honorific title given to pilgrims (*see also Hajji*).

Hajji: pilgrim. An honorific title given to those who have completed the *Hajj*.

halal: all that is lawful, as decreed by Allah. The basic maxim is that 'all is allowed save that which is prohibited'.

hammam: communal bathing area, particularly common in Turkey. Also used to refer to the toilet/bathroom in some Arabic countries.

haram: all that is unlawful or prohibited by Allah.

imam: religious teacher. Also used to describe the one who leads the daily congregational prayers.

Iqamah: the second call to prayer immediately preceding the prayer itself.

Iqra: to read. The first word of the Qur'an to be revealed.

Islam: literally the act of submitting oneself to the will of Allah through a conscious and voluntary act. The religion of the Muslims.

istinja: washing one's genitals with free-flowing water after urinating or evacuating. An essential prerequisite before the daily prayers.

jalb al-maslahah: a term from the Islamic legal system which refers to the ethical principle of the accruement of benefit.

Ka'bah: The Sacred Mosque in Mecca, Saudi Arabia, towards which Muslims will face in their daily prayers.

makruh: something that Islam strongly discourages, but does not forbid.

malb: the very essence of a thing. Used to denote both the physical and metaphysical heart. Derived from the verb *taqalaba* meaning 'to turn'.

mandub: a recommended religious duty; a course of conduct which earns moral reward if followed; however, a person who does not follow such a course of conduct is not open to punishment.

Maslahah: benefit, particularly in relation to public interest considerations.

miswaak: a tooth-stick commonly used in many parts of the Muslim world.

mubah: an act permitted by Islamic Law but having no religious value or significance.

mufsidat: refers to corrupting drugs.

muraqqidat: anaesthetics, drugs which anaesthetise the five senses completely.

muskirat: refers to intoxicants, which inebriate and cause a feeling of excitement and well-being.

Muslim: one who has freely and consciously submitted to the will of Allah.

Namaz: used by Muslims from the Indian subcontinent for *Salah* (*see below*).

Qiblah: the direction of The Sacred Mosque in Mecca.

Qur'an: Allah's final revelation to Man, and the primary source of Islamic Law. Previous revelations have included The Psalms of David, The Torah of Moses and The Gospel of Jesus.

Ramadan: the ninth month of the Islamic calendar and the month in which all adult Muslims are required to fast. Fasting involves a complete abstinence from food and drink and sexual intercourse during daylight hours. An exemption exists for the elderly, the infirm, and menstruating, pregnant or lactating women.

Sabr: steadfastness, resilience, fortitude, patience and gratitude to Allah at all times, and in all situations.

Salah: the obligatory prayer performed by Muslims five times a day.

salim: one who is healthy (from *salama* meaning safety).

salla'Llahu alayhi wa-sallam: the sending of salutations on the Prophet. An appendage used by the devout whenever they make mention of Muhammad.

Sawm: fasting during the month of Ramadan. An obligation for all sane, healthy adults.

Shahadah: the testimony of faith: 'There is no deity other than Allah; Muhammad is the Messenger of Allah.'

Shariah: the moral, social and legal code of Islam. The primary sources of Shariah are the Qur'an and the body of Prophetic teachings comprising the *Sunnah* (*see below*).

Shifa: a cure or healing. One of the attributes of Allah is *as-Shafi* meaning 'The Supreme Healer'.

Shi'is (plural *Shi'a*): distinguished from the mainstream community after the Prophet's death on the basis of their conviction that his descendants alone should be the successors to his temporal authority and that these descendants are protected from committing sins.

Sufi: pursuing a spiritual path under the direct guidance of a Master.

Sunnah: literally, a way or path. The pattern of conduct of the Prophet Muhammad comprising his sayings, practices and sanctioned customs.

Sunni: the main body of Muslims representing over 90% of the total Muslim community.

Tahneek: the Prophetic practice of rubbing a small piece of softened date into the upper palate of the newborn.

tahsiniyyat: the comforts are those matters which add to the joy and experience of life and are in the nature of desirabilities as they seek to attain refinement and perfection in the customs and conduct of people at all levels of achievement.

Taweeez: an amulet containing prayers or sections from the Qur'an.

tayammum: dry ablution involving symbolically wiping the hands and face with dust; a dispensation for those in whom the more usual wet ablution (*see Wudu*) is problematic or may be injurious to health.

Ulema: literally, 'the learned'. Those chosen by the community and charged with the responsibility of formulating Islamic Law using the principles enshrined within the Qur'an and Sunnah.

Umrah: a 'lesser' Pilgrimage to The Sacred Mosque performed outside of the *Hajj* season.

wudu: ritual ablution that precedes the daily canonical prayers. Involves washing, in sequence, the hands, face, arms and feet.

Zakat: alms tax made payable by all those who have savings above a minimum level at the rate of 2.5% on annual savings.

Index